The Ultimate
ALKALINE
Lifestyle & Detox

For Health & Glowing Skin

Dr. Anna Brilli
https://alkaglow.com/

Copyright © 2024

All rights reserved.

All rights reserved. No part of this publication may be reproduced, distributed, or transmitted in any form or by any means, including photocopying, recording, or other electronic or mechanical methods, without the author's prior written permission, except in the case of brief quotations embodied in critical reviews and certain other non-commercial uses permitted by copyright law. For permission requests, please get in touch with the author.

Endorsements

"Dr. Anna Brilli's book offers a brilliant, complete, and detailed way to know the importance of keeping our body away from the dangerous acidic state behind the systemic inflammation that leads to numerous chronic diseases with undesirable ends. Her expert analysis and recommendations are vital in modern times where an increase of commercial "junk" food products become a temptation for our taste but poisonous for our health, and our incompetence to respond appropriately to environmental stress is collecting taxes on our organisms. Give yourself the unique possibility of reading a book that will take you to the sanctuary for sound health."
Dr. Luciano A. Pulido, Ph.D., DNM - International speaker on Quantum Consciousness, Mind, and Holistic Health, and author of the book "The Black Hole Syndrome of Human Consciousness: A Critical Analysis Turning Disease into Health and Frustration into a Successful Life."

"The ultimate Alkaline lifestyle book by Dr Anna is amazing. It's changed how I see food and especially what I eat. Her knowledge is profound, she will change you and better your body!"
Vishal Madhani - Director & Physiotherapist, West 1 Health, London, UK

Sönd
View more at **sondskin.co.uk**

Table of Contents

INTRODUCTION
We promise, we get it.. 1
Why did we create this book?.. 2
A welcome from Dr. Anna Brilli... 3

UNDERSTANDING WHAT HAS BROUGHT YOU HERE
A 'normal' state of feeling under par... 7
The problem with modern life.. 8
Could homeostasis be the answer?... 9

INTRODUCING THE ALKALINE LIFESTYLE
Alkalinity & pH... 11
Are we healthiest in an alkaline state?.. 12
An introduction to the alkaline lifestyle.. 14
The elements of an alkaline lifestyle.. 15
Happiness is a journey.. 18

THE SEVEN DAY DETOX
Kickstarting your alkaline lifestyle with a detox............................ 20
Your 7 day detox plan.. 24
Your detox shopping list... 26
Your detox week is about to start.. 28

DAY EIGHT AND ONWARDS
Day eight - what's next?... 31
The golden rules... 34
The power of positivity & letting go... 36
Alkaline forming foods.. 39
Acidic forming foods... 42

Sönd
View more at sondskin.co.uk

Alkaline Nutrition

The alkaline approach to nutrition **47**
Understanding food intolerances **50**
The alkaline diet and hormones **52**
Are you chewing your food correctly? **54**
What our stool reveals about our health **57**
Empowering heavy metal detoxification **59**

UNDERSTANDING INGREDIENTS

Going green...with your diet **63**
Demystifying gluten **66**
Everything you need to know about sugar **68**
Dairy vs non-dairy - making the switch **73**
Embracing healthy fats **76**
The hidden dangers of low-fat and fat-free foods **78**

DRINKS

Why water is the key to health **81**
The impact of our morning coffee fix **85**
The health impact of tea **88**
Alcohol: Understanding the Impact and Choosing Wisely **90**
The bitter truth of soft drinks **92**
Hidden dangers of energy drinks **94**
The dynamics of fruit juices **96**

SHOPPING

Being mindful of the seasons **98**
Decoding food labels **101**
Buying and storing different ingredients **103**

THE ALKALINE KITCHEN

The alkaline kitchen **107**
Cooking methods for an alkaline lifestyle **110**

SUPPLEMENTS

The requirement for supplements.. **113**
The healing potential of sea-derived supplements................................ **115**
The health benefits of brown algae.. **117**

ALKALINE SKINCARE

The power of alkaline skincare... **121**
Dry brushing.. **123**
Eliminate toxins with an alkaline bath... **124**
Daily lymph drainage exercises... **126**
Algae-based facial treatments... **128**
Algae-based body treatments... **130**

ALKALINE LIFESTYLE

An important daily routine... **133**
The benefits of a cold shower.. **134**
The importance of good quality sleep.. **137**
Mastering a good breathing technique.. **140**
Breathing techniques that benefit health... **143**
The importance of exercise... **146**
Biofilia for vitality and wellbeing.. **148**
Biofilic harmony with nature... **150**
The dark side of blue light... **152**
An important note.. **155**

DETOX WEEK PLAN, SHOPPING LIST & RECIPES

7-Day detox meal plan.. **157**
Your Detox shopping list... **158**
Alkaline vegetable stock... **160**
Carrot, coriander & sesame Seed soup.. **162**
Popey Chia Soup... **163**
Tomato & Basil Soup.. **164**
Green Artichoke & Bean Soup... **165**
Pesto Green Soup... **166**
Asian Detox Soup.. **167**
Green Garden Lime Soup.. **168**
Cream of Peas Cold Soup... **169**
Purple Cream Cold Soup... **170**
Cucumber & Grass Cold Soup... **171**
Avocado Dream Cold Soup.. **172**
Asparagus Cold Soup... **173**
Gazpacho... **174**
Vichyssoise... **175**
Red Juice... **176**
Green Juice... **177**
Coco Tea.. **178**
Lemon Tea... **179**

POST DETOX ALKALINE SOUP RECIPE

How to make a soup.. **181**

REFERENCES   **183**

We promise, we get it

You've probably tried everything under the sun to achieve the health and glowing, clear, dewy looking skin we all aspire to.

You're probably tired of hearing that feeling comfortable in your own skin is the key to confidence, because, let's face it, that's easier said than done when dealing with skincare issues that take their toll day-to-day.

We know all about it because we help people with non-conformist skin every single day.

The skin serves as a mirror reflecting our overall health, especially the condition of our gut and intestines. That's why it's crucial to focus on maintaining a healthy body, as it directly contributes to a radiant and glowing complexion. By nurturing our internal health, particularly our gut and intestines, we can positively impact the appearance and health of our skin, promoting a natural and vibrant glow.

You have to change what you are doing to see change.

If you've been struggling for a long time, we know how exhausting it can feel to keep trying. Please know that we have worked hard to make this as easy to commit to as possible, and you don't have to do everything perfectly to see great results.

Our approach isn't complicated; it will take a little getting used to, but ultimately, it involves small changes, one step at a time.

Allow us to introduce ourselves...

We're Sönd, and we help our customers achieve healthy, feel-good skin and overall wellbeing.

Our approach is unusual, which is why it works when other approaches haven't.

The power of alkalinity

Created to give your skin some TLC without the fuss, we use the ancient power of alkalinity and some thoroughly modern science to create a no-nonsense skincare routine that turns sensitive or acne-prone skin from a daily worry into something you don't need to think about.

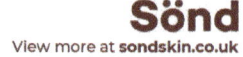

Why did we create this book?

Here at **Sönd**, we are on a mission to free people from the prison of non-conformist skin.

We know what it feels like to have given up relying on your skin.

While our skincare products deliver amazing results for our customers, we know that skin is built from the inside out. So to have healthy, happy-looking skin, we need our bodies to be healthy.

One of the most important elements of having a healthy body is feeding it the nutrients it needs not only to survive but to thrive.

That's why we've worked with the incredible **Dr. Anna Brilli** to create this book which will show you how to fuel your body to produce healthy, glowing skin.

Give yourself the knowledge you need to make the required changes

Many factors impact our health and skin. The way we live, the food we eat, the stress levels we expose ourselves to, and the list goes on.

This book has been designed to give you an insight and understanding of the significant factors that impact your health and skin.

This will hopefully allow you to stop feeling lost and give you the knowledge you need to start making the required changes to reach your health and skin goals.

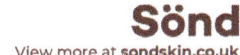

A welcome from Dr. Anna Brilli

Hello and welcome to your first step towards taking a holistic approach to getting clear, brighter-looking skin. Thank you for taking the time to read this book. I hope you get as much value from it as I did writing it.

Medical Consultant and Holistic Nutritionist

I have over 35 years' experience as a Medical Consultant and Holistic Nutritionist and I'm a registered member of the International College of Holistic Medicine (ICHM) and a proud member of the British Holistic Medical Association (BHMA).

Using my qualifications, extensive experience, and a lot of curiosity, I've developed my alkaline-based approach to natural wellbeing.

What began as an interest in the processes of ageing and metabolism led me to conduct thorough research into the lesser-known causes of premature ageing, poor metabolism, obesity, skin conditions, sleep disorders, and chronic inflammatory diseases.

Questioning the norm

Modern medicine is without doubt a marvel, but my research led me to wonder about a couple of things.

Could we be managing some of these common lifestyle problems holistically?

Could our body have the potential to heal itself without the use of chemicals?

I've discovered that the answer to both of these questions is 'yes'.

Maximising health

Most of us are unaware that we can heal ourselves naturally, and my goal is to maximise my clients' own health by using the power of their own bodies to boost their immune systems. And now I want to share that wisdom with you.

Find out more about Alkaglow

If you would like to find out more about me and my alkaline concept, you can visit www.alkaglow.com

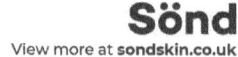

A holistic, alkaline methodology

My holistic, alkaline methodology helps to slow down the ageing process, increase physical strength, improve mental clarity, and resolve skin concerns.

I use a variety of techniques depending on the health problem I'm working with. These techniques include nutritional assessment and detox plan, alkaline skincare, and breathing exercises.

Through my methodology and embracing my alkaline-based approach to natural wellbeing, my clients have successfully changed their lifestyles to live healthier, happier, and more fulfilling lives.

And now it's your turn. Your body is a natural pharmacy, and it already holds the power to change. By simply adjusting your intake and quality of food, water, vitamins, and minerals, your body is entirely capable of healing itself from within.

Are you ready? Then let's begin.

Dr. Anna Brilli
Alkaline Nutritionist & Health Coach

Dedication

I dedicate this book to my lovely daughter, Sonia, who has been my constant companion and a great source of support throughout my journey in founding the alkaline lifestyle.

Her presence and assistance have been invaluable, and I am grateful for her unwavering encouragement as I embarked on this path.

Together, we have explored and embraced the principles of the alkaline lifestyle, and I hope this book will inspire and guide others to embark on their own transformative journey towards a healthier and more balanced life.

With all my love,
Anna

Understanding What Has Brought You Here

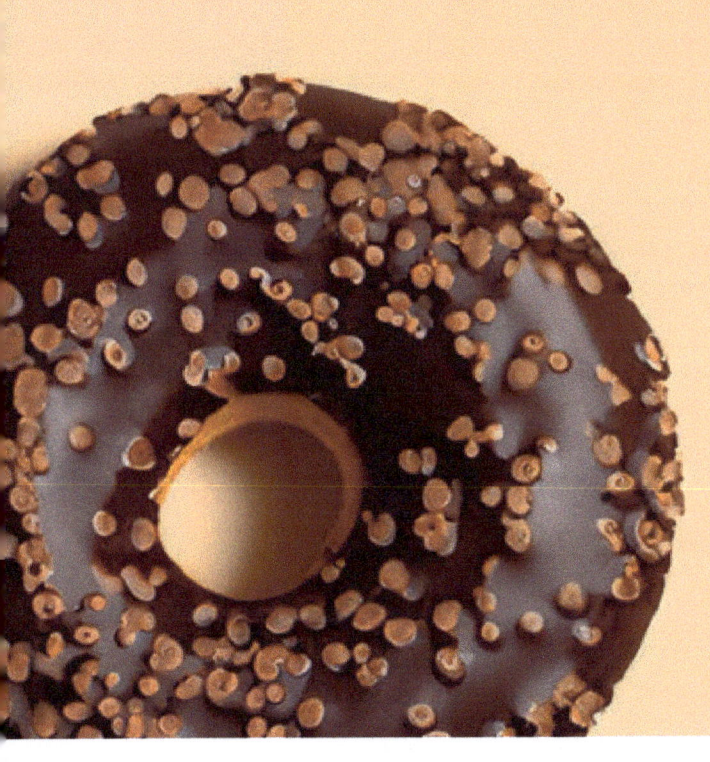
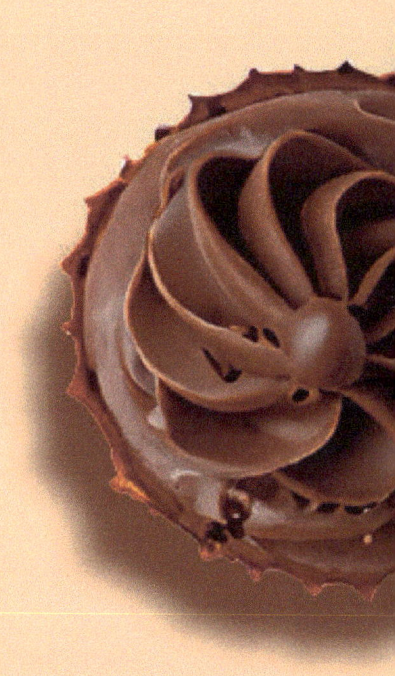

Sönd
View more at **sondskin.co.uk**

A 'normal' state of feeling under par

Is feeling lethargic, with no get up and go, zero physical energy, misbehaving skin, acne breakouts, body aches and pains and brain fog, just, well, normal, for you?

It is for many of us. But feeling that way shouldn't be our norm, nor does it have to be.

According to the World Health Organisation (WHO), health is a "state of physical, mental and social wellbeing".

But there are so few truly healthy people on the planet. Why? I think it's because of people's stressful lives and the foods they eat.

The human body is perfectly assembled for living. Yet despite this perfect assembly, we've made ourselves ill because we've disturbed the relationship we once had between us and nature.

Being ill should not be a normal part of living.

The most important discovery we can make is to know that we can reset everything. There are numerous teachings about living a healthy life in harmony with nature, and there is no teaching that is as comprehensive as living an alkaline lifestyle.

But what exactly is an alkaline lifestyle?

To understand that, we need to first understand the impact modern life has on our diet, lifestyle and wellbeing.

Go to the next section to find out more.

The problem with modern life

In some way, all of us are affected by the hectic rhythms of everyday life. Stressful, busy lives mean that we make decisions based on being time- and cost-effective. This leads us to make choices that are good for us in the short term but may have long-term consequences for our health.

The pace of life has changed

The food industry has tapped into our modern fast paced lives and has drastically changed our eating habits by encouraging us to eat time-rich, nutrient-poor, refined, and packaged foods. This type of diet simply doesn't have the capacity to provide our bodies with the nutrition we need and instead creates an ongoing inflammatory process. In the long term, this inflammation can contribute to the development of chronic diseases, misbehaving skin, and weight gain.

Sedentary lifestyles

Due to the rapid advancement of technology and changes in our social lives over the last few decades, our lifestyles have dramatically changed. The majority of our time is now spent in front of a computer, TV, or telephone screen, and the amount of time we spend sitting down has drastically increased.

Higher stress levels

As a population, we're also accustomed to high stress levels, which lead us to make poor decisions regarding the health of our food and to use 'crutches' such as alcohol and drugs. This then serves to create malnutrition and intoxication, which then leads our bodies to live in an acidic state rather than an alkaline one.

Industrialisation

In the past century, we've seen an enormous expansion of the chemical industry. Pesticides, fertilisers, preservatives, growth hormones, antibiotics, and flavour enhancers are all now rife, meaning that literally everything we draw from the natural world for our existence—air, water, and food—is contaminated with a cocktail of chemicals, contributing to the acidic state within our bodies.

All of the above factors promote an acidic lifestyle that creates an accumulation of toxins in the internal and external cellular spaces that block the proper functioning of the cells and the communication between them, which can lead to various diseases. But other factors as part of a busy, modern lifestyle also lead to illness and disease.

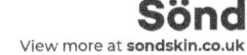

Could homeostasis be the answer?

Based on many years of research and study about our biological systems, it became obvious that the most important aspect of good health is our body balance, or state of homeostasis.

Homeostasis is the body's natural way of balancing everything, including our gut bacteria, hormones, blood cell production, immune system, temperature, and crucially, our pH.

The moment any of these elements are put out of balance by factors such as the Western diet, a lack of sleep, stress, fast food, sugary drinks, alcohol, or smoking, we experience health issues.

These can range from fatigue, digestive problems, compromised microbiota, weight management, skin concerns and problems with mental clarity.

"I believe that if we supply the body with what it needs to maintain balance, everything will change."

-Dr. Anna Brilli

Why is alkalinity important?

Our body, as the perfect bio-machine, always tries to maintain its fine balance, or homeostasis.

A fundamental aspect of this balance is maintaining the body's natural pH, ideally 7.365, which is slightly alkaline.

Adopting an alkaline lifestyle that includes a well-balanced and varied diet can help prevent most modern diseases, such as obesity, heart disease, and type 2 diabetes.

Skip to the next chapter to find out more about what alkalinity is and the benefits it can bring to your health.

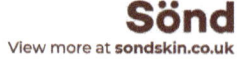

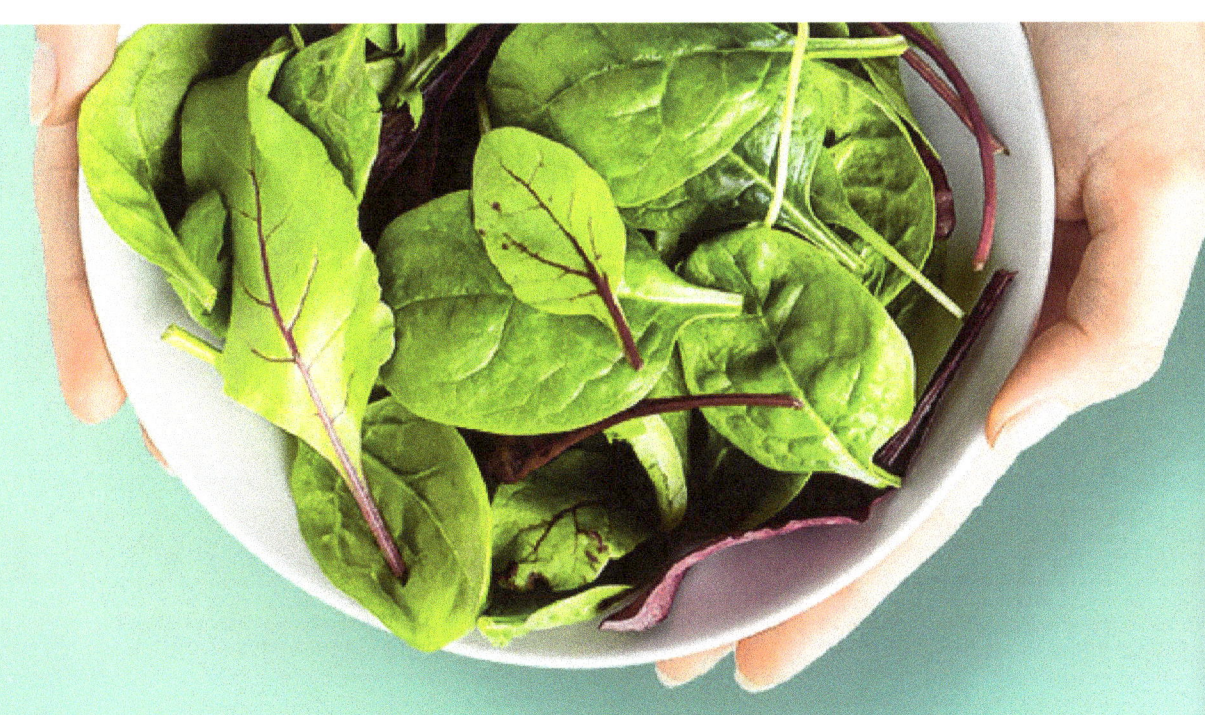

Introducing The Alkaline Lifestyle

Alkalinity & pH

Alkalinity is a measure of pH and is opposite to acidity.

The pH scale ranges from 0 to 14.

Acids are at the low end of the pH scale, from pH 1 to 6, with 1 being the most acidic, and alkalis are at the higher end of the pH scale, from pH 8 to 14, with 14 being the most alkaline.

A pH of 7 is considered neutral.

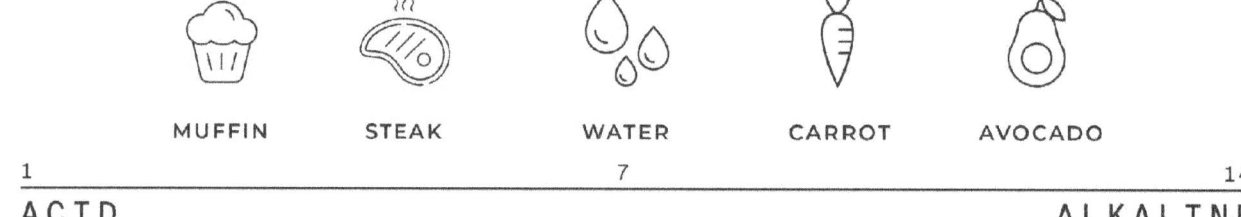

Are we healthiest in an alkaline state?

Our bodies require a slightly alkaline environment with a pH of 7.365 to ensure optimal health and functioning.

Let's take a closer look at why our bodies benefit from an alkaline environment:

Cellular vitality

Cells thrive in a slightly alkaline environment. Many essential cellular processes, including enzyme activities and nutrient uptake, function best within specific pH ranges. An alkaline environment promotes efficient cellular metabolism and overall vitality.

Acid-base balance

An alkaline environment helps counteract the effects of excessive acidity in the body, a condition known as acidosis. Acidosis can disrupt cellular functions and weaken the immune system, making it essential to maintain proper pH levels.

Bone health

Balanced pH levels are vital for strong bones. When the body becomes overly acidic, it may draw minerals like calcium from bones to restore pH balance. This process can weaken bones and increase the risk of osteoporosis.

Detoxification support

Optimal pH levels facilitate the body's natural detoxification processes. An alkaline environment aids in the elimination of waste and toxins, reducing the strain on organs responsible for detoxification, such as the liver and kidneys.

Immune System Resilience

Pathogens and harmful microorganisms find it harder to survive in an alkaline environment. By maintaining an alkaline pH, the body creates a less hospitable environment for these invaders, bolstering the immune system's defenses.

Inflammation Management

Chronic acidity can contribute to inflammation, a root cause of various health issues. An alkaline environment helps regulate inflammation, promoting a healthier internal state.

Sustained energy

Balanced pH levels contribute to efficient cellular metabolism, which translates to sustained energy levels. An alkaline environment supports the body's energy production processes, aiding in improved vitality.

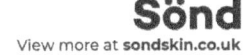

View more at sondskin.co.uk

Digestive harmony

A slightly alkaline gut environment supports optimal digestion. It encourages the activity of digestive enzymes and fosters the growth of beneficial gut bacteria, leading to improved nutrient absorption and digestive health.

Internal acidosis can lead to skin breakouts and irritation

When our bodies are too acidic, our cells can't perform their required functions to stay healthy, which can show on our skin.

This can manifest in skin breakouts, irritation, and sensitivity.

In essence, by creating an alkaline-friendly internal environment, we provide our bodies with the ideal conditions for the body's natural healing mechanisms to thrive and maintain excellent health.

An introduction to the alkaline lifestyle

My alkaline-based approach to natural wellbeing has the power to change the way you feel. It can help to boost your energy levels, improve your mental clarity and gut function, reduce inflammation and give you clearer skin.

An alkaline lifestyle is a holistic and innovative approach to personal wellbeing with the awareness that our own health is influenced by us and the life we lead.

Can you change the pH of your body?

Yes, it is possible to influence your body's pH. Studies have shown that performing certain breathing exercises can increase your body's pH. While this is true, following an alkaline lifestyle isn't about increasing your pH.

As we covered earlier, the majority of our body is slightly alkaline with a pH of 7.365, and the body does all it can to keep this balance. If you have an acidic lifestyle, eat acidic food, and are under chronic stress, it puts a lot of pressure on your body to counteract this. This can lead to inflammation and in turn health and skin issues.

So living an alkaline lifestyle is about reducing the stress on your body to allow it to perform at its best.

Living an alkaline lifestyle encourages us to become aware of the biochemical acid-alkaline balance within the body and how it's essential to our well-being. It's a natural way of living designed to achieve total well-being, a healthy weight, happy, vibrant skin, good immunity, and an excellent quality of life. Essentially, an alkaline lifestyle means nurturing a healthy internal and external environment.

In an ideal world, an individual would opt for such a lifestyle long before suffering illness and disease. However, it's never too late to start living an alkaline lifestyle.

Go to the next lesson to find out how to support your body's natural alkaline state for optimal health.

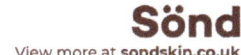

The elements of an alkaline lifestyle

There are simple techniques that can be practiced every day that help to reduce acidity levels and create a more alkaline environment for your body to live in.

Everything we cover here in this section will be dealt with in more detail later on in the book.

Diet

Did you know that 70% of our immune system is based in our gut? If we're not feeding our bodies the best nutrition, we won't be able to keep our bodies healthy. Highly processed foods are linked with inflammation, which can lead to a variety of health issues as well as irritated skin and flare-ups.

In order to keep our skin clear and happy, an alkaline, low-inflammation diet filled with nutrients is best. This means eating fresh, whole foods and ingredients as much as possible and keeping highly processed foods to a minimum.

Reducing or eliminating the intake of foods that trigger intolerances is key to managing symptoms and preventing associated inflammation. If food intolerances are suspected, it's advisable to consult a healthcare professional or a registered dietitian to determine the culprits and develop an appropriate dietary plan to alleviate symptoms and reduce inflammation.

Breathing

Among the most well-known of these techniques are respiratory and breathing exercises. These are fundamental, as they help to restore and alkalise the body fluids. By maintaining alkalinity through breathwork, we're able to change our gut microbiome, which, apart from having other health benefits, also directly determines serotonin levels. Serotonin is our happy hormone. Therefore, with higher serotonin levels and an improved mood, we can more easily change our lifestyle and eating habits. A virtuous cycle!

Fresh air

Our spaces should be well-ventilated, and we should aim to be outside in the fresh air as often as possible each day.

Spending time and doing physical activity in nature, offers an irreplaceable source of strength, which helps better breathing and circulation overall.

Water

Water is essential for the functioning of the human body, yet not all water is created equal.

Sadly, water pipes are chemically treated, and some bottled water may lack stringent regulations, leading to potential contaminants or lower quality compared to regulated tap water.

Alkaline water is rich in minerals and ions, so it's best to use alkaline water filters to ensure you are drinking water that is optimised for your health.

Cosmetics

Many of the products we apply to our skin get absorbed into our body and can impact our pH balance. Our skin's connective tissue should have a pH of around 7.3; if we apply acidic products to our skin, they can get absorbed and affect this important balance.

Therefore, it's best to aim for cosmetics and beauty products that are natural and free from alcohol and chemical preservatives, and choose a natural deodorant over an antiperspirant. Also aim for natural cleaning products and natural candles and diffusers that add fragrance to the home.

Movement and activity

Apart from dietary errors and the harmful effects of stress, an additional enemy to our body that can cause disease, weight problems and skin concerns is a sedentary lifestyle.

Doing any kind of activity, compatible with your physical strength and age is fundamental to activating the movement of the lymphatic system, metabolic processes, blood circulation, cell oxygenation, and reducing fat mass, which, if high, has been shown to slow down the metabolism in the first place.

Managing stress

One of the most common causes of weight gain and chronic lifestyle diseases is stress. Various scientific studies have confirmed that stress stimulates the production of cortisol, a hormone that gives us the strength to overcome our problems. However, if the quantity of cortisol is too high for too long, our body receives the signal to accumulate fat in the abdominal area, also known as visceral fat, which is the most dangerous and hardest to eliminate.

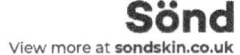

Environment

The development of civilization has its advantages, but it's brought with it an increase in electromagnetic radiation that hangs around in the environment. The earth's natural magnetic fields aren't dangerous to humans and have a certain positive effect on the proper function of our body. However, technical devices such as mobile phones, wifi, antennas, radios, headphones, neon bulbs, microwave ovens, and much more have negatively affected the environment our bodies live in. Therefore, their use should be reduced to what is necessary.

The environment in which we live should be simple to allow the flow of energy. Spaces should have enough natural light, and they should be filled with natural colours. As all colours emit waves of different wavelengths, it's a good idea to represent all colours of the spectrum in our living and working spaces.

Sleep

It's important for us to allow our bodies a minimum of six to eight hours of good-quality sleep per night. This is vital for maintaining the levels of a protein hormone called leptin. Leptin is responsible for the management of our appetite and metabolism and for the production of melatonin, which in turn is responsible for strengthening the immune system and protecting the central nervous system.

If all this sounds daunting, don't worry

This book will guide you through all the dos and don'ts of an alkaline lifestyle and will help you through a seven-day alkaline reset that will do wonders to help you on your way.

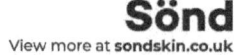

Happiness is a journey

Remember that happiness is a journey, and embracing an alkaline lifestyle can be a positive step towards improving overall well-being.

Be patient with yourself and allow time for adjustments and improvements. By making conscious choices that support your health and happiness, you can create a more fulfilling and joyful life.

Each day, take small steps towards enriching your life, and watch as these actions gradually weave themselves into your daily routines.

Remember, it's not about achieving perfection in one giant leap, but rather the consistency of making positive changes, no matter how small they may seem. Celebrate each effort you make, knowing that with time and dedication, they will transform into meaningful habits that shape your life in profound ways.

Believe in yourself, and let every day be a testament to the incredible strength and resilience within you.

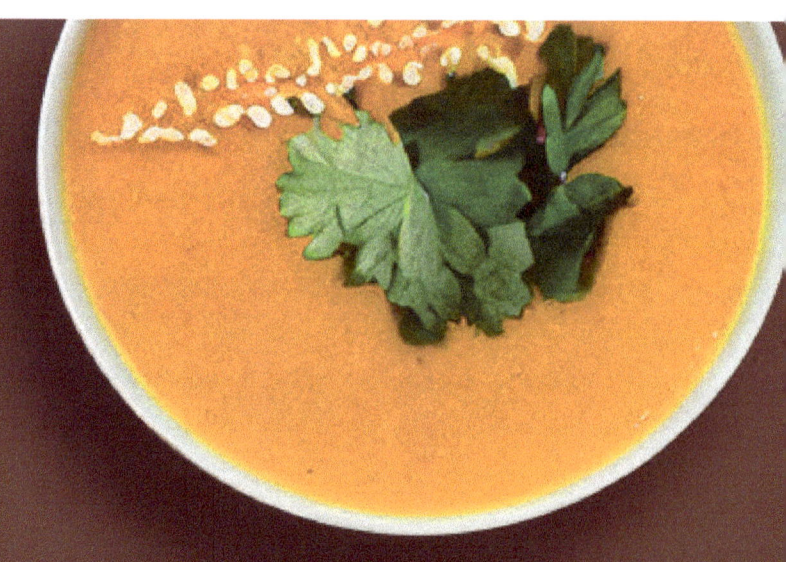

The Seven Day Detox

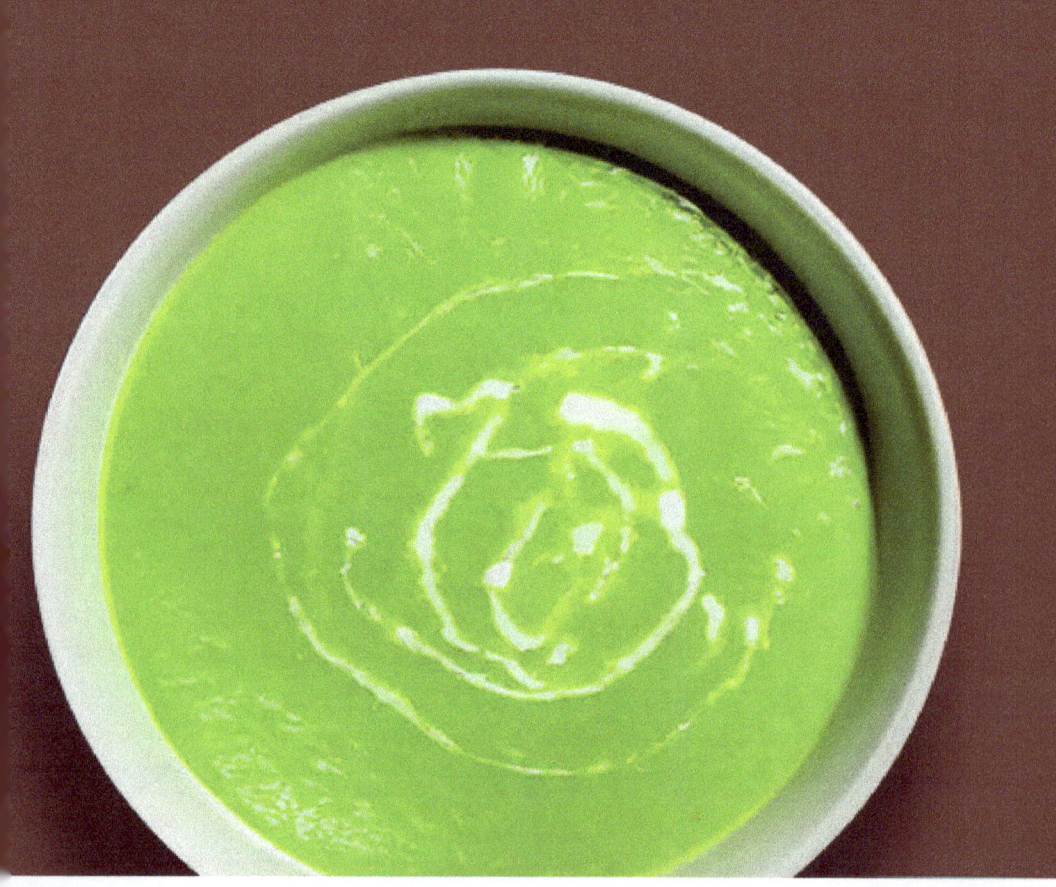
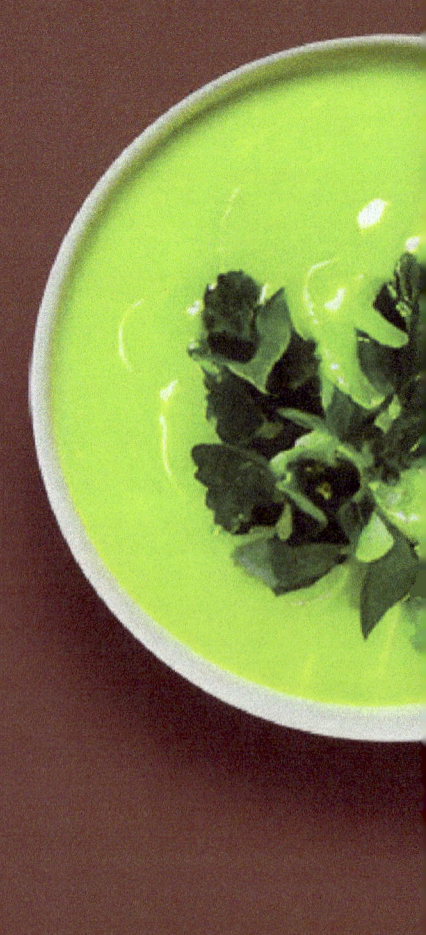

Kickstarting your alkaline lifestyle with a detox

Join me on my seven-day alkalising detox to rebalance and reset your body so that it's ready for great things. The next seven days may feel challenging, but trust the process and enjoy the journey both right now and beyond.

The aim of the detox

An alkaline detox isn't about mindlessly increasing the pH of the body from the lower acidic range of pH values to the higher alkaline ones.

Instead, it assists the body in maintaining its homeostasis and finding its sweet spot of pH 7.356 without adding stress or fatigue.

Having an acidic body state places excessive stress on the organs.

This then leads to an overproduction of the stress hormone cortisol, which itself leads to insulin resistance, an increase in visceral fat cells (the fat that sits around the organs), and inflammation.

Chronic inflammation, that is, inflammation that's been hanging around for a while as a result of mainly diet and stress, is the leading cause of lifestyle diseases such as obesity, type 2 diabetes, and heart disease.

Add to this an impaired ability for the body to deal with oxidative stress caused by free radicals (nasty unstable molecules of oxygen caused by stress, a poor diet, an unhealthy lifestyle, smoking, and environmental pollutants), and we're facing a lot of health issues and even speeding up our natural ageing processes.

Acidity, inflammation, and oxidative stress are our enemies. But all is not lost.

My seven day alkalising detox will prepare your body for a long-lasting, effortless alkaline lifestyle and will provide you with all the vitamins, minerals, chlorophyll, antioxidants, fibre, good fats, and protein that your body needs to feel nourished, cleansed, healed, and repaired.

A focus on liquids

During your seven-day detox, you'll only be consuming liquid food, including soups, vegetable juices, teas, and plenty of water.

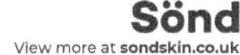

Despite this sounding quite extreme, I've designed this alkaline detox to feed your body with all it needs to rebalance, repair, and rebuild.

Rest and reset your digestion

Consuming only liquids requires very little energy for digestion, absorption, and assimilation of nutrients, helping to give your digestive organs a rest and reset, allowing them to recover from any fatigue.

At the same time, the beneficial nutrients you'll be consuming will support your body to eliminate toxins, promote rest and recovery, reduce inflammation, and flood your body with antioxidants.

Here's some useful information on the why and how of my alkalising detox:

- Consuming only liquids for seven days helps to give your digestive system a rest and allows for easier absorption of nutrients.
- It contains nothing but real food and real nutrients that support the body and all its organs while your internal pH is rebalanced.
- Consuming vegetables in liquid form means that meals are more nutrient-dense and increase the quantities you're able to consume in one sitting.
- Fresh, liquid nutrients help to rebalance, rebuild, repair, alkalise, fight inflammation, and neutralise free radicals.
- The immune, digestive, endocrine, detoxification, and acid-buffering systems all benefit the most from a seven-day alkalising detox.
- The detox shouldn't leave you feeling hungry, but if you do (and you've drunk more alkalising water to check you're not thirsty instead), then feel free to consume more of the liquid foods that form part of this detox.
- At the end, you'll feel physically and emotionally lighter, with a healthy, positive attitude and a good mood.

The goal

The main goal of this detox is to restore balance in the body and support it in its endeavours to maintain the constant balance, or homeostasis, of pH as well as heart rate, and the production of enzymes, hormones.

All this, as well as keeping the immune system healthy, maintaining the balance of good and bad gut bacteria, and fighting free radicals—what an exhausting job! The body does all this without being asked; the least we can do is spend seven days helping to reset all of these systems.

Because if this delicate balance is lost, we become tired and unwell, develop pain and inflammation, gain weight, experience a lack of sleep, and much more. It's for this reason that we need to give our bodies the right tools to function properly without adding additional stress.

The Five Golden Rules when carrying out my seven day detox:

1. No fruit
2. No sugar
3. No gluten
4. No coffee
5. No alcohol

You should also drink a minimum of two to three litres of alkaline water per day.

During detox week, you may experience symptoms that are common with any detox. These include:

- Headaches
- Dizziness or lightheadedness
- An upset stomach
- Spots and acne breakouts
- Light flu-like symptoms

Many people experience no symptoms, but if you do, they should only last from a few hours to a couple of days. They are caused by toxins leaving the system through urinating, defecating, perspiring, and breathing.

The best time of year to complete this detox is in the spring, with a repeat in the autumn and, if possible, once again after the Christmas and New Year period of excess.

Are you ready to start the seven day alkalising detox to rebalance and reset your body so that it's ready for great things?

The next seven days may feel difficult, but trust the process and enjoy the journey both right now and beyond.

Important note

The detox plan I offer is a safe program that can be followed for up to two weeks.

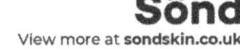

Here's to your vibrant health and renewed vitality, as you embrace the **1-week Alkaline Detox Lifestyle** through the art of nourishing meals!

Your 7 day detox plan

Take a look now at my Seven Day Detox Meal Plan in the recipes section at the back of the book. You'll see seven meals for each of the seven days of the detox.

These are my suggestions, but feel free to make some tweaks if there are certain juices or soups that don't work for you at those times. You can always remove ingredients, but don't be tempted to add any that aren't already mentioned here as they could be acid-forming, which is defeating the object of this detox.

You'll notice that many of the soups are repeated during the week so it's completely ok to make them in large batches and keep them in a sealed container in the fridge for two to three days.

The juices are more susceptible to spoilage and losing vitamins, so only store these for up to two days, and always in a tightly sealed Thermos flask away from light, air and warmth.

Once you've planned your seven day detox, sticking closely to my example you'll want to know how to create all of these delicious drinks, juices and soups so here's how!

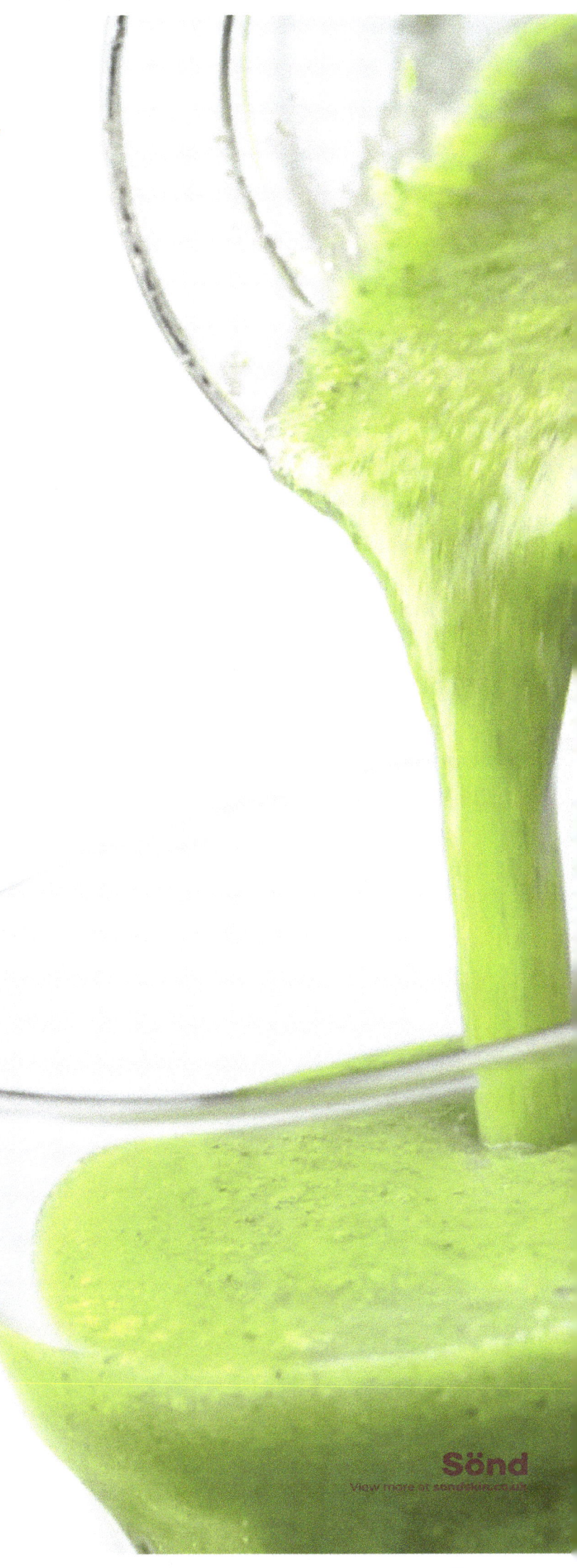

For an energising and alkalising detox, follow this well-rounded schedule.

Upon waking

Start your day with a cup of tea.

Before breakfast and mid morning

For a nutritious and alkalising boost, opt for a fresh juice, you can choose from the vibrant red juice; alternatively, try the green one.

These juices will provide essential vitamins, minerals, and antioxidants to kickstart your day with vitality.

Breakfast

For a refreshing and light breakfast, enjoy a cold soup.

These cold soups will nourish your body and keep you hydrated.

Mid afternoon

Sip on more fresh juices in the mid afternoon to maintain your energy levels and support your alkaline lifestyle.

Feel free to choose from the previously mentioned red and green juices.

Lunch and dinner

For both lunch and dinner, indulge in a variety of delicious and nutrient-packed soups from the plentiful selection of recipes provided.

Each soup is carefully crafted with alkaline vegetables, herbs, and spices to support your seven day detox and overall well-being.

Throughout the day

Stay hydrated and refreshed by drinking plenty of alkaline water. Aim for at least two to three litres daily to help flush out toxins and maintain proper hydration.

By following this detox schedule, you'll nourish your body with alkalising and nutrient-dense liquids, allowing your digestive system to rest and recover. The abundance of vitamins, minerals, and antioxidants will support your body's natural detoxification processes, promoting overall health and well-being.

Remember to listen to your body and adjust the recipes to suit your dietary needs, ensuring a successful and enjoyable detox journey.

Cheers to a revitalised, alkaline lifestyle!

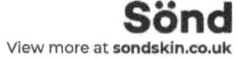

Your detox shopping list

Preparing for a detox is key so that you have everything you need ready for when you start, meaning that you don't have to improvise or make sacrifices that may make you stray from your detox plan.

You will find your shopping list in the Detox Recipes section at the back of this book.

Choose your "day one" wisely

For this reason, I usually advise making Sunday "day one" of your detox.

You can make Saturday your shopping day so that you don't have to rush around looking for out-of-stock ingredients, preparing your soups and juices, and getting everything ready.

Starting a day during the working week can cause stress and overwhelm, as, let's face it, we all run out of time.

If you work shift patterns or don't fit into a regular Monday to Friday working week, then you can obviously adapt your start day to suit you.

Split your shopping

That said, I also advise splitting your shopping lists into two: one for the first half of the week and the other for the second half.

This ensures that all your ingredients are as fresh as possible. So, it will involve a trip to the shops or the market midweek, but by then you'll be in full swing, and it shouldn't be as stressful or as overwhelming.

Also, you'll already have all the store cupboard ingredients, such as seeds, salt, and nuts, from the first shopping list, so the second trip will see you bringing home fewer bags.

Fresh ingredients

If you look at my example Seven Day Detox Meal Plan, you'll see that as the week goes on, I introduce new soup recipes, the ingredients for which need to be super fresh.

I've designed my example shopping lists to reflect the ingredients you'll need for days 1 to 4 and then days 5 to 7.

If you've personalised this and deviated slightly from mine, then you can easily personalise your shopping lists too. (You can remove ingredients that you're not keen on, but don't add any others that aren't on your detox shopping list.)

Find your detox groove

For this shopping list, I've tried to stick to the right quantities for one person to follow the seven day detox.

It's a rough guide, however, so if you need more or less of each ingredient, go for it; you'll soon find your detox groove anyway. Remember, you shouldn't feel hungry, but if you do, simply increase the quantities of the juices and soups you're consuming.

Quality over quantity

An alkaline lifestyle doesn't have strict portion sizes; it's all about the quality of the ingredients, not the quantity.

Plus, the products you buy now will see you through your detox, and then they'll become a significant part of your future alkaline lifestyle.

Don't forget to take along your reusable shopping bags!

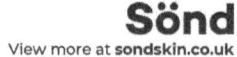

Your detox week is about to start

Ready to embark on your alkaline journey? Let's get started with your detox week! Step by step, we'll make positive changes together. Embrace the process and experience the transformation towards a vibrant, healthy, and happy life.

As you embark on this transformative week, don't focus on perfection. Embrace every small step you take towards positive change, and celebrate each moment of growth. Let go of any guilt or self-judgment, for every choice you make is an opportunity to nourish your body and mind.

Throughout your detox week, stay connected with your body's signals. Listen to what it craves, and observe how it responds to different foods and activities. Be mindful during meals and savour the flavours and textures, knowing that each bite contributes to your well-being.

Incorporate the detox teas, juices, and soups as suggested, but feel free to make some adjustments to suit your preferences and needs without adding any food that is not on the detox list.

Remember, it's not about rigid adherence but rather creating a sustainable and balanced routine that aligns with your unique journey.

Stay attuned to the changes within yourself as the week progresses. Notice the increased energy, the lightness in your step, and the clarity of your mind. These are all signs that your body is thriving in an alkaline environment.

Surround yourself with positivity and support throughout this process. Share your experiences with your friends, colleagues, and loved ones. Connecting with like-minded individuals can provide encouragement and inspiration during your journey.

As you proceed, let go of any fear or doubt. Trust in yourself and your body's innate wisdom to guide you towards what feels right. With each passing day, you'll become more in tune with your alkaline lifestyle, and it will become a natural extension of who you are.

Embrace this transformative time, and remember, it's a journey, not a destination. Be gentle with yourself, and allow room for growth and exploration. There may be moments of challenge, but also moments of triumph, all of which contribute to your evolution.

So, take a deep breath, and with a heart full of joy, begin your detox week.

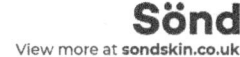

You have everything you need within you to create a beautiful and alkaline life. Embrace this new chapter with lots of courage and excitement, and let it lead you towards a vibrant and harmonious existence.

Wishing you an empowering and transformative detox week on your alkaline journey.

With love and support,
Anna

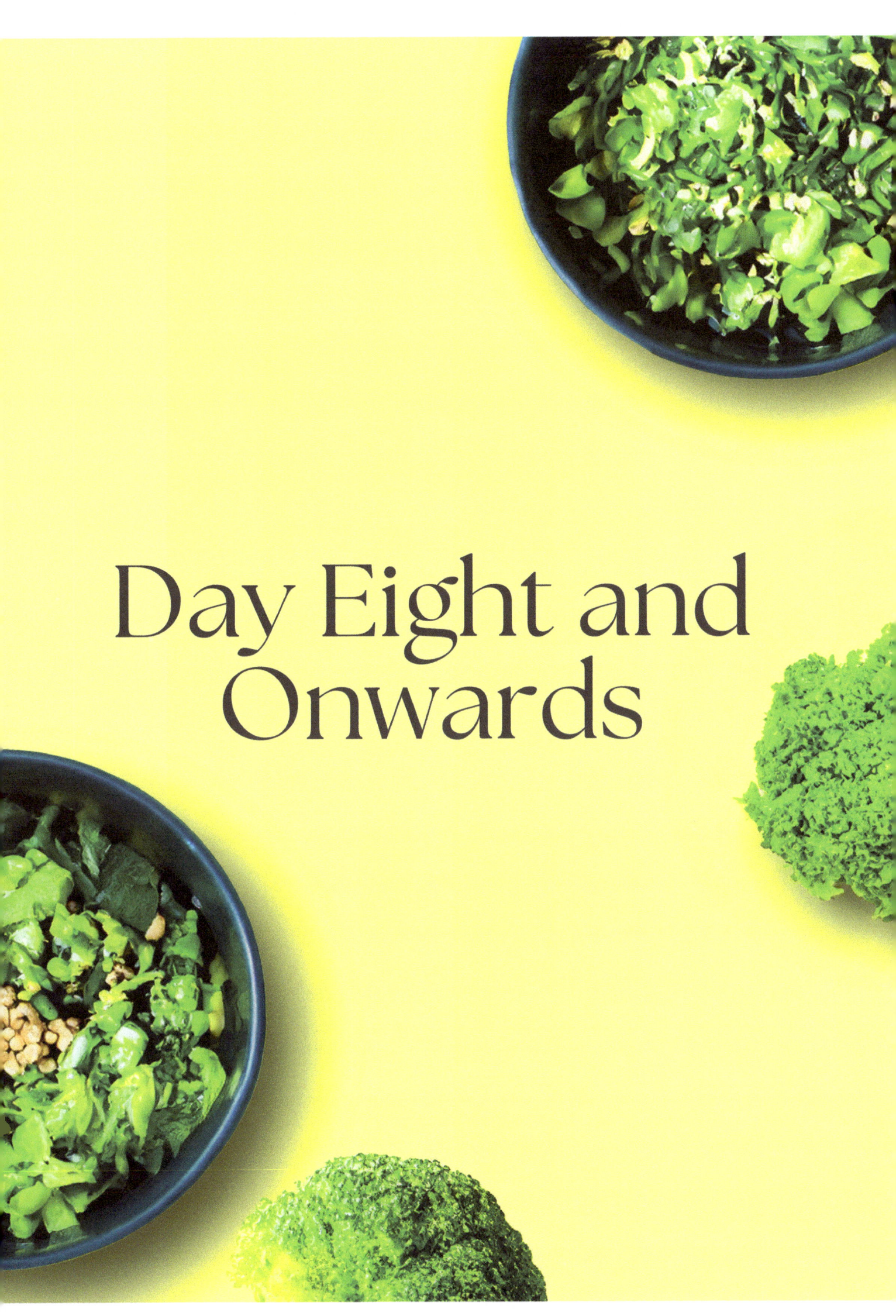

Day Eight and Onwards

Day eight – what's next?

So, you've woken up on the morning after the week before—your detox is finished. Well done!

You may have noticed that you feel less slow and sluggish and that your afternoon lethargy has disappeared, along with any sleep difficulties, brain fog, and trouble concentrating.

You may also notice that your skin feels clearer and brighter, and your mood is uplifted. Aches and pains may have long gone, and you may have even lost a few pounds and inches.

You really are on the cusp of something amazing; what's not to love?

But what do you do now?

You can go back to the old ways, right?

No! It's crucial that you don't undo all that hard work, and actually, I suspect that you feel so good today that you won't want to slip into bad habits anyway.

Today really is the beginning of the rest of your life, feeling light, bright, healthy, happy, full of vitality, and energised. It feels good, doesn't it?

Taking an 80:20 approach

If we make healthy choices the majority of the time and then let go a little every now and again, there's no reason why we have to completely give up the foods we might enjoy that don't fit into the alkaline way of eating and living.

So I'll repeat what I said at the beginning: I'm not advocating strict diets, guilt cycles, or surviving on little more than lettuce. Nor am I advocating a strict, narrow, uninspiring diet.

I'm advocating the notion of 80:20, eating alkaline foods 80% of the time, with 20% left over for non-alkaline foods that won't then override all the good work you're doing for the majority of your week.

For many people, craving all those acid-forming foods they've just avoided for a week is completely normal. So don't feel like a failure if this is you. But I urge you to try not to give into the cravings, as you've come so far and done so much good.

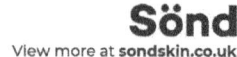
View more at sondskin.co.uk

A crossroads

Day eight really is day one of living your new alkaline life, and today presents an important crossroads: do you turn around and go back on yourself and eat the diet that made you feel so sluggish, tired, unwell, and unhappy before? Or do you take the road ahead, towards a happy and healthy life? It's not a tough question when we put it like that, is it?

I think you should choose the road ahead. But you knew that anyway.

Helpful dos and don'ts for today

Follow the guide below just for today and see how it feels, and then maybe you'll do it tomorrow too. And the next day, and the day after that...

Do:
- Always start the day with a detoxifying lemon or cocoa tea.
- Keep up with a morning juice to start the day with an invigorating antioxidant boost.
- Hold off cooked, solid food until lunch if you can; if not, Introduce a solid breakfast and chew again at breakfast; porridge oats and quinoa cold pudding are great, or avocado on organic rye bread or gluten free brown bread is great. You can also add some hemp seeds or almond flakes on top.
- If you eat meat, fish, and dairy, add a little of these foods to your lunch or evening meal, but get the majority of your protein from beans, pulses, lentils, and chickpeas (remember to stick to the 80:20 rule if you do eat animal protein).
- Make your own soup using alkaline vegetables three times a week for lunch or dinner.
- Add a green salad to each meal.
- Continue to drink 2 to 3 litres of water a day, more if you feel you need it, especially since you'll be consuming fewer liquid foods than you did during your detox. It's crucial to understand that when we're thirsty, we may mistake it for hunger, so when you feel hungry, drink a full glass of water and wait ten minutes. Are you still hungry? If not, you were probably thirsty.
- Carry on adding extra virgin olive or avocado oils to your food to ensure you're consuming enough good quality omega-3 oils.
- Add as much anti-inflammatory ginger and turmeric to your diet as possible, or take a good quality curcumin supplement.

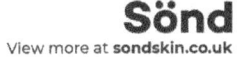

Don't:
- Give in to your cravings; you might feel like you're missing out on certain foods, but your body really isn't.
- Consume refined sugar.
- Consume gluten, or try to reduce it to a minimum.
- Eat refined white carbohydrates, processed, junk, or packaged food.
- Restart drinking coffee; choose matcha green tea instead.
- Completely avoid dairy if you don't want to; you can eat goat cheese or yogurt occasionally if you like.

Living an alkaline lifestyle takes less effort than doing your seven day detox. That was simply to kickstart your body into feeling and looking better.

Now, you'll be able to indulge in some of the foods you're missing, knowing that 80% of the time, you're treating your body to what it needs.

If you're struggling with cravings, know that they won't last forever. (If they do, nibble on some raw vegetables, almonds, or cashews.)

In fact, most cravings are over in 20 minutes, so find something to do, such as read or go for a walk, to take your mind off things. Or use a mindfulness app to listen to an urge surfing meditation and surf the wave of the urge to give in to your cravings. And don't forget, you may be thirsty, so drink a glass of water, wait ten minutes, and see if you're still hungry.

Eventually, you will really reach the point where you think, *"I really don't want to put junk food, processed food, and too many other acid-forming foods into my body."* When you get there, it'll feel incredible.

Stick to the 80:20 rule of eating 80% alkaline foods and 20% acid-forming foods, and your physical and emotional health will continue to benefit now and long into the future.

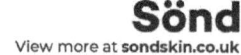

The golden rules

By now, you've probably got a pretty good idea of what it means to live an alkaline lifestyle. But it's still a good idea to recap, so I've put together some golden rules (including some new ones that we haven't touched on yet).

You can use this list as a quick reference if you're unsure of anything after you've detoxed and are embarking on your new alkaline lifestyle. For more details on any of the items below you can refer to the relevant chapter in this book.

Diet

Diet is the most important factor in living an alkaline lifestyle. What we eat and how we fuel ourselves have a profound effect on our overall health and well-being.

- Aim for a diet that's 80% alkaline and 20% acid-forming foods every day.
- Consume home-cooked, fresh food and avoid calorie-dense, nutrient-poor, pre-packaged, and pre-cooked foods with any questionable ingredients.
- Never skip breakfast; a red or green juice is ideal.
- Consume seasonal, locally grown vegetables, and choose organic as much as possible.
- Spinach is amazing; add it to all the juices and meals that you can.
- Eat some raw vegetables every day.
- Eat a green salad with each meal.
- Keep animal-based proteins such as meat, fish, eggs, and dairy to a minimum and opt for plant-based proteins in the form of beans, pulses, lentils, and chickpeas instead.
- If you eat animal products, consume them at lunchtime to give your body time to digest them. If you eat them in the evening, try to eat them at least two hours before bed.
- Avoid eating fried food.
- Keep gluten and refined sugars to a minimum, ideally working towards completely eliminating them.
- When you eat fruit, eat the whole fruit rather than juicing it, as juicing removes the fibre and makes the fructose (fruit sugar) more available (which goes directly to the liver where it can cause inflammation).
- Fruit makes an excellent snack, but it should not be eaten close to your main meal. Aim for just one piece (no more) of low-sugar, alkaline fruit per day.
- Decrease the number of times you use the oven to cook food; choose raw as much as possible.
- Avoid using a microwave to cook or reheat your food; use a saucepan on a hob instead.

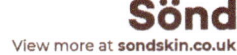

- If you're eating out, eat some raw vegetables before you go.
- Eat mindfully at each meal, chewing each mouthful slowly and purposefully between 32 and 52 times, and put your cutlery down in between each mouthful.
- Avoid distractions from the TV, reading material, and your smartphone when eating; make your only focus your food.
- Sit up straight at a table when eating each meal, and don't rush.

Drink

How and what we choose to drink and hydrate our bodies with will have an impact on how energised we feel, both physically and emotionally.

- Drink a minimum of 2 to 3 litres of room temperature alkaline water each day.
- Avoid drinking water with meals; instead, drink two glasses of water before each meal.
- Drink a red or green juice every morning, but don't add any fruit.
- Drink a detoxing lemon or cocoa tea as soon as you wake up.
- Reduce your caffeine intake to one coffee a day, preferably none.
- Avoid fizzy drinks (even diet ones), fruit juices, or ice cold drinks.
- Limit your alcohol intake, and if you do drink alcohol, try to stick to red wine that's high in polyphenols and antioxidants.

Lifestyle

Our habits and behaviours have a significant impact on our wellbeing, and we should place as much importance on these, as our diet.

- Practice deep breathing exercises for 2 to 3 minutes before each meal.
- Learn how to truly breathe properly and practice this three times a day (morning, midday, and before bed) for five minutes each time to balance your blood pH levels, boost your energy, and settle your nervous system.
- Exercise at least three times a week; this can be a long walk or a light jog.
- Take good quality vitamin and mineral supplements base on your needs. It is best to speak to a qualified nutritionist to create a personalised plan for you.
- Aim to be asleep each night before midnight, sleep for at least 6 to 8 hours each night, and don't use your mobile phone when you're in bed.
- Finally, think positive, and you'll be positive!

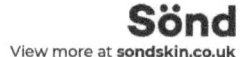

View more at sondskin.co.uk

The power of positivity & letting go

Having a positive attitude and the ability to let things go are crucial elements in maintaining a healthy and balanced life.

Letting go of negativity and embracing a positive mindset can significantly impact our overall well-being and contribute to an alkaline lifestyle.

Here's why:

Positive thinking can improve our mental health by reducing stress, anxiety, and depression. When we let go of negative thoughts and focus on the positive aspects of life, we cultivate resilience and emotional strength.

Studies have shown that a positive attitude can have a positive impact on physical health. It can boost the immune system, lower blood pressure, and improve cardiovascular health.

By letting go of stress and negative emotions, we can create a healthier internal environment.

A positive attitude fosters better relationships with others. It promotes empathy, understanding, and effective communication, leading to healthier and more fulfilling connections with friends, family, and colleagues.

Letting go of grudges and negative emotions frees up mental and emotional energy. This newfound energy can be redirected towards productive and positive activities, making us more efficient and focused in our daily lives.

Life is full of challenges, but a positive attitude helps us face them with greater resilience. When we let go of setbacks and focus on solutions, we become better equipped to overcome obstacles and emerge stronger on the other side.

Positive thinking allows for clearer and more rational decision-making. By letting go of fear and doubt, we can approach decisions with a balanced perspective and make choices that align with our long-term goals.

When we let go of negative emotions, we create space for emotional balance and inner peace.

This emotional equilibrium is vital to navigating life's ups and downs with grace and composure.

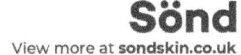

An alkaline state of mind

Incorporating a positive attitude and the ability to let go into our daily lives complements the principles of an alkaline lifestyle. It aligns with the goal of creating a harmonious and balanced internal environment. Just as we strive to maintain a healthy pH balance in our bodies, we should also cultivate positivity and release negativity to achieve an alkaline state of mind.

So, let us embrace positivity, practice gratitude, and learn to let go of what no longer serves us. By doing so, we open ourselves up to a world of possibilities, enhanced well-being, and a deeper appreciation for the beauty of life.

Remember, positivity is a choice we can make every day to nurture our bodies, minds, and spirits and to live our lives to the fullest.

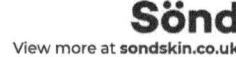

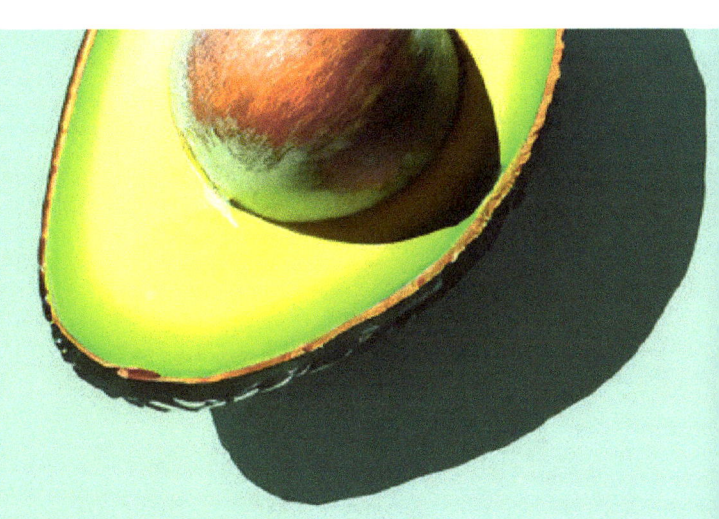
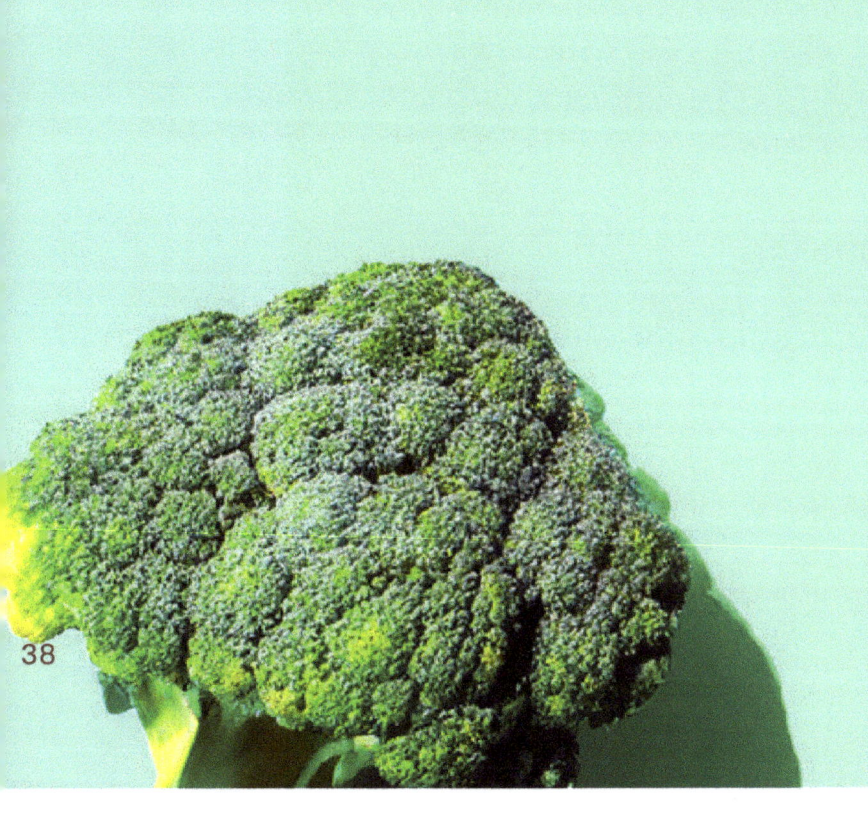
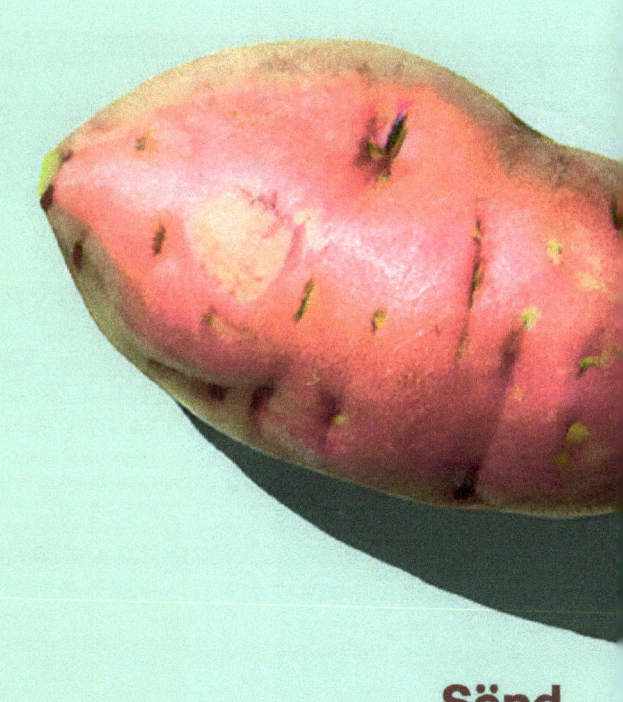

Alkaline & Acidic Forming Foods

Alkaline forming foods

Vegetables

A — ASPARAGUS - ARTICHOKE - AUBERGINE

B — BASIL - BEETROOT - BROCCOLI - BRUSSELS SPROUTS

C — CHARD - CUCUMBER - CABBAGE - CARROT - CAULIFLOWER - COLLARD - CAPSICUM - CORIANDER - CHIVES - CHILLI - CELERY - COURGETTE

D — DANDELION

K — KALE

L — LETTUCE - LEEKS

N — NEW POTATO

O — ONION - OKRA

P — PARSLEY - PEAS - PUMPKIN

R — RADISH - ROCKET - RHUBARB

S — SWEET POTATO - SPINACH

W — WATERCRESS - WAKAME

Alkaline forming foods

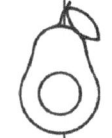

Alkaline Fruit

AVOCADO - BANANA - COCONUT - FIGS - GRAPEFRUIT - LIME - LEMON

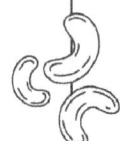

Alkaline Nuts & Seads

ALMONDS, CASHEW NUTS - CHESTNUTS, SUNFLOWER, SESAME, LINSEED, PUMPKIN SEEDS, CHIA SEEDS

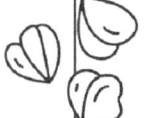

Alkaline Sprouts, Cereals & Beans

AMARANTH, BUCKWHEAT - BROAD BEANS - FENUGREEK - GREEN MUNG BEANS - KAMUT - LENTILS - LUPINS - MILLET - QUINOA - RICE (BROWN) RED BEANS - SOY BEANS - WHITE BEANS

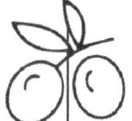

Alkaline Oils

AVOCADO OIL - OLIVE OIL - LINSEED OIL - BORAGE OIL

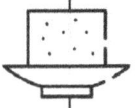

Alkaline-Friendly Milk and Dairy

GOAT MILK - TOFU - ALMOND MILK

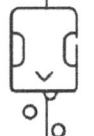

Alkaline Sweeteners

STEVIA

Alkaline forming foods

Alkaline Drinks

MACHA ROOT - ALKALINE WATER - HERBAL TEAS & INFUSION

Acidic forming foods

The foods below are all acid-forming once consumed, so should take up no more than 20% of your diet. Remember that no foods are forbidden, it is just about finding a balance where your body is still able to function and perform it's required prodcesses.

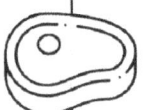

Meat

DUCK - LAMB - BISON - SEA BASS - RABBIT - BOAR - PHEASANT - BEEF - MUTTON - PORK - GOOSE - CHICKEN - BACON - HAM - SAUSAGE - SALAMI - TURKEY - VEAL

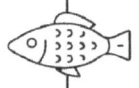

Fish

LOBSTER - SQUID - MUSSELS - SCALLOPS - CRUSTACEANS - CRAB - SHRIMPS - SNAIL / ESCARGOT - COD - OYSTER - SEA BREAM - OCTOPUS - STURGEON - REDFISH - SALMON - SARDINES - CEVICHE - SOLE - TUNA - TROUT

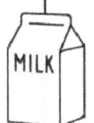

Dairy & Eggs

BUTTER - CASEIN - ICE CREAM - MILK - SOUR CREAM - WHEY - YOGURT

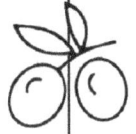

Oils

PEANUT OIL - CANOLA OR OTHER VEGETABLE OILS - SUNFLOWER OIL - MARGARINE - WALNUT OIL - SESAME OIL

Acidic forming foods

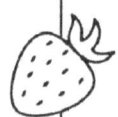

Fruits

APRICOT - ORANGE - PINEAPPLE - WATERMELON - BERRIES - CANTALOUPE - CHERRY - CHESTNUT - DATES - STRAWBERRY - RASPBERRIES - MANGO - MELON - APPLE - MANGOSTEEN - CRANBERRIES - POMEGRANATE - NECTARINE - PEACH - PEAR - PLUMS - PLUM - PAPAYA - CURRANTS - GRAPES - RAISINS

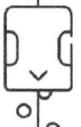

Sweeteners

CANDIES - ARTIFICIAL SWEETENERS - FRUCTOSE - HONEY - MALTITOL - MOLASSES - MAPLE SYRUP CORN SYRUP - AGAVE SYRUP - MAPLE SYRUP - YACON SYRUP - SACCHARIN - SORBITOL - SUCRALOSE - XYLITOL - COCONUT SUGAR - SUGAR

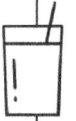

Drinks

ALCOHOL - SPARKLING WATER - TAP WATER - FLAVOURED WATER - CARBONATED DRINKS - DECAFFEINATED DRINKS - ENERGY DRINKS - COFFEE - PASTEURISED FRUIT JUICES - BLACK TEA

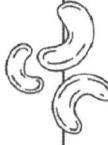

Nuts

PEANUTS - CHESTNUTS - HAZELNUTS - BRAZIL NUTS - MACADAMIA NUTS - PECANS - PISTACHIOS

Acidic forming foods

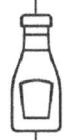

Dressings

VINEGAR (INCLUDING BALSAMIC) - KETCHUP - MAYONNAISE - SOY SAUCE - MUSTARD - PICKLES TABASCO - TAMARI - WASABI

Bread, pasta and more

BISCUITS - BREAD (WHITE) - CHIPS - CRACKERS - CHOCOLATES - MUSHROOMS - YEAST - MISO NOODLES - PIZZA - PASTA (WHITE) - RICE (WHITE)

Alkaline Nutrition

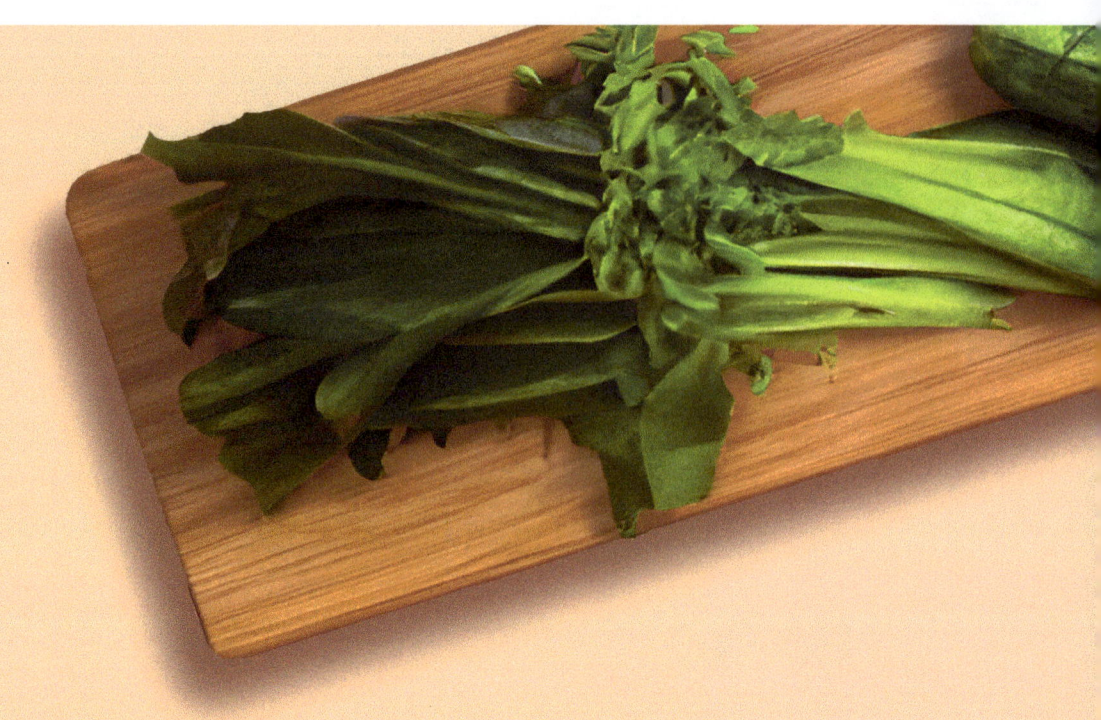

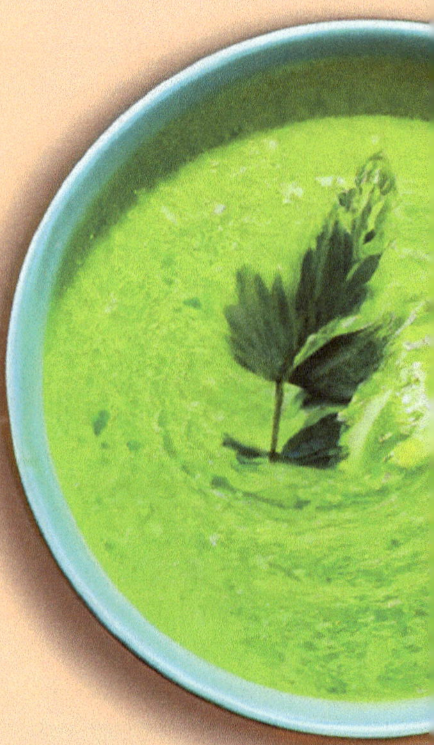

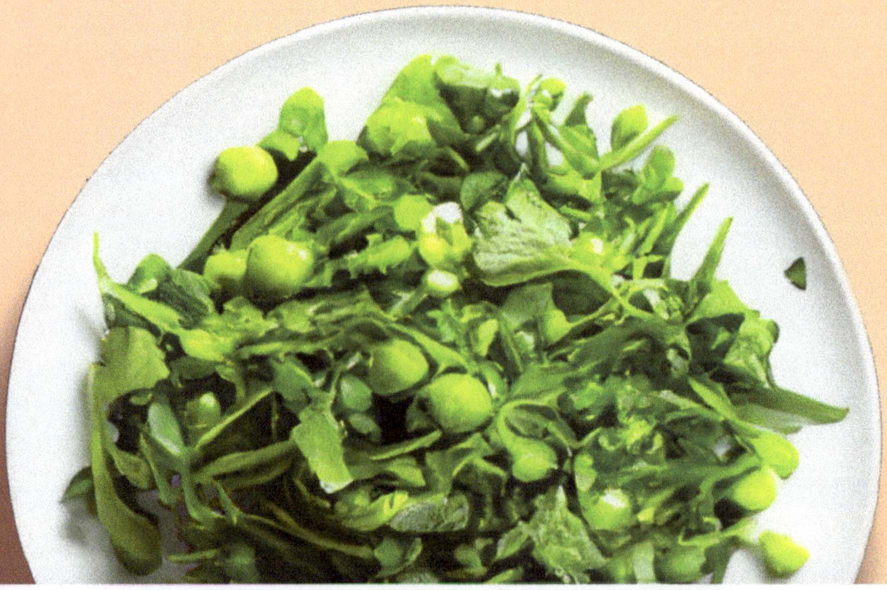

Welcome to a transformative culinary experience, where the rejuvenating essence of an **Alkaline Diet awaits.**

The alkaline approach to nutrition

Living the alkaline lifestyle is exactly that—it's a lifestyle that, with practice, will become second nature. It isn't a strict diet, with hard and fast rules and immovable goal posts.

I personally believe that placing harsh dietary restrictions on our lives doesn't get us far; it simply serves to make us develop cravings that eventually become so strong that we bend the "rules" and then enter a crazy cycle of bingeing and guilt. So you most definitely don't have to suddenly overhaul your diet, give everything up, survive on salads, and eat perfectly every single day (or from day one).

Phew! Now that you've breathed a huge sigh of relief that achieving a healthier, happier, more fulfilling life doesn't mean living a miserable existence, we can talk about maintaining clarity and focus.

Our relationship with food should be positive. Food is used to celebrate success, milestones, life events, birthdays, and anniversaries. Having an indulgent treat should be filled with joy, not guilt. When living an alkaline lifestyle, we can still enjoy this positive relationship with the things we choose to eat.

We don't have to secretly have "cheat" days or meals that "reward" us for "good" behaviour. This is toxic and negative and uses food as a bartering tool when it should simply be enjoyed. Food should be cherished for nourishing our bodies and allowing us to go to sleep each night without feeling hungry.

If we make healthy choices the majority of the time and then let go a little every now and again, there's no reason why we have to completely give up the foods we might enjoy that don't fit into the alkaline way of eating and living.

So I'll repeat what I said at the beginning: I'm not advocating strict diets, guilt cycles, or surviving on little more than lettuce. Nor am I advocating a strict, narrow, uninspiring diet. I'm advocating the notion of 80:20: eating alkaline foods 80% of the time, with 20% left over for non-alkaline foods.

Following an alkaline lifestyle isn't a 'diet'. Instead, it is what it says: a lifestyle. When you dig deeper, it makes sense: alkaline foods are natural, unprocessed, and high in antioxidant, anti-inflammatory nutrients.

Once you begin the alkaline way of eating, you'll learn that alkaline foods are delicious anyway! They're full of health-promoting nutrition and flavour, and they're far from boring or faddy.

Alkaline living and eating will fill you with energy, still allow you to have fun with your food, be social, and give your body the nourishment it needs to flourish with health and vitality.

It means being in tune with your body, listening to what it needs, and giving it what it needs. When you become familiar with alkaline eating, you'll know that there's no stress over what you can and can't eat. Instead, I'll provide you with everything you need to make the right decisions.

The effects of eating acid forming foods

When we eat acid-forming foods such as refined sugars, animal proteins, and hydrogenated fats, the body quickly enters stress mode. We might not notice it, but behind the scenes, the body releases cortisol, and the gut releases hydrochloric acid. The body, therefore, needs to work hard to recreate an alkaline environment.

In the short term, this is okay. We might treat ourselves to ice cream on a hot day, and the natural capacity we have to buffer the acids will help to correct the balance. But we only have a limited buffering capacity. If we constantly eat an acidic diet, the body is in a constant state of stress.

When we've reached our acid buffering capacity, the body turns to other ways of maintaining its slightly alkaline pH. This includes drawing calcium from the bones and producing more and more cortisol, leading to weakened bones, reduced immunity, inflammation, insulin resistance, and problems with the gut.

In the long term, an acidic state can lead to chronic adrenal fatigue, weight gain, skin problems, digestive problems, rheumatoid arthritis, and chronic inflammation. The longer the imbalance lasts, the more stable and progressive the course of the disease.

An alkaline diet supports our health

The most important thing we can do to help our organs work with less fatigue and to maintain our optimal pH level is to change our eating habits.

The alkaline diet isn't 'faddy' or asking you to do anything out of the ordinary.

It simply focuses on health-giving, nutritious foods that don't ask your body to adjust simply to digest them.

What are acidic or alkaline diets?

An acidic diet is one that is high in fat, animal protein, sugar, and salt. Conversely, an alkaline diet is rich in plants, vegetables, olive oil, and oily fish. It is filled with nutrients, vitamins, and minerals that fuel the body and support the health of the body and mind.

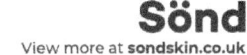

Follow the simple 80:20 approach

I advocate an 80:20 approach: aim to eat an alkaline diet 80% of the time, allowing 20% for treats that won't override all the good work you're doing for the majority of your week.

Look at all the things you can eat, rather than the ones you can't

If understanding what you need to reduce in your diet is causing you overwhelm or anxiety, then look at my lists as a way of incorporating more of the things that form part of an alkaline diet. These small adjustments and looking at things from the perspective of what to easily add rather than stressfully thinking about what to remove will help ease you in.

In the long term, this will mean a better chance of success and a gradual process of successfully removing the majority of the acid-forming foods currently in your diet.

Learning to understand your behaviour

But what about if I have a "bad" day and things all go wrong? I hear you cry! We're all humans, and humans don't get everything right all of the time.

If you do have a day or longer where you're neglecting alkaline foods in favour of acid-forming ones, think about why. Are you stressed, upset, or hurting? Or were you in a celebratory mood or on holiday?

Taking a moment to understand your own personal 'why' (and notice how it makes your body feel) will help you to make changes and get back on track, rather than emotionally beating yourself up and slipping further and further into a downward spiral.

Don't forget, what you eat will give your body what it needs to not only survive but also thrive. Or it can give your body things that promote inflammation and disease. The choice is yours, and I know that since you're here, you're choosing to thrive.

So listen to your body, find your groove, and allow it to maintain its perfect pH balance for health and vitality. You hold the power to do so!

Remember that happiness is a journey, and embracing an alkaline lifestyle can be a positive step towards improving overall well-being. Be patient with yourself and allow time for adjustments and improvements. By making conscious choices that support your health and happiness, you can create a more fulfilling and joyful life.

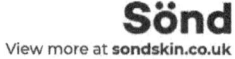

View more at sondskin.co.uk

Understanding food intolerances

Food intolerances occur when the body has difficulty digesting certain foods, leading to various uncomfortable symptoms. Unlike food allergies, which involve the immune system's response to specific proteins in foods, food intolerances typically involve difficulties in breaking down specific food components, such as carbohydrates, sugars, or additives.

When someone has a food intolerance, the digestive system may react adversely to certain foods or ingredients, leading to symptoms like bloating, gas, abdominal pain, diarrhoea, or nausea. In some cases, food intolerances might also trigger inflammation.

The mechanism behind how food intolerances can lead to inflammation varies depending on the specific intolerance.

Lactose Intolerance

People with lactose intolerance lack enough lactase, the enzyme needed to break down lactose (a sugar found in milk). Undigested lactose can ferment in the gut, leading to the production of gases and causing abdominal discomfort. Prolonged exposure to undigested lactose might irritate the intestinal lining, potentially leading to low-grade inflammation in the gut.

Gluten Sensitivity

In some individuals, sensitivity to gluten, a protein found in wheat, barley, and rye, can lead to symptoms akin to celiac disease but without the immune system's involvement. The consumption of gluten might cause digestive issues and trigger an inflammatory response in the gut.

Histamine Intolerance

Some people have difficulty breaking down histamine found in various foods like aged cheese, cured meats, and fermented foods. The accumulation of histamine in the body due to poor breakdown can result in symptoms resembling an allergic reaction and might also contribute to low-grade inflammation.

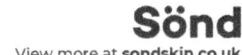

View more at sondskin.co.uk

Persistent exposure to foods that one is intolerant to can lead to chronic, low-grade inflammation in the digestive system. This inflammation may affect the gut lining and contribute to conditions like irritable bowel syndrome (IBS) or other gastrointestinal issues.

Reducing or eliminating the intake of foods that trigger intolerances is key to managing symptoms and preventing associated inflammation. If food intolerances are suspected, it's advisable to consult a healthcare professional or a registered dietitian to determine the culprits and develop an appropriate dietary plan to alleviate symptoms and reduce inflammation.:

The alkaline diet and hormones

The alkaline diet is often promoted as a way to achieve better health by maintaining a slightly alkaline pH level in the body. While the scientific evidence supporting the direct influence of the alkaline diet on hormones is quite limited, some aspects of the diet may indirectly impact hormone balance.

Let's explore how the alkaline diet may affect various hormones in the body:

Insulin

The alkaline diet encourages the consumption of vegetables, and whole grains while discouraging refined carbohydrates and sugary foods.

Through the promotion of a lower intake of high-glycemic foods, the alkaline diet may help regulate blood sugar levels and reduce the need for excessive insulin secretion.

Cortisol

Chronic stress can lead to increased cortisol levels, which can disrupt hormone balance and impact various bodily functions. The alkaline diet, rich in fruits, vegetables, and antioxidants, may help combat oxidative stress and inflammation, contributing to better stress management and potentially reducing cortisol levels.

Leptin and ghrelin

Leptin and ghrelin are hormones involved in appetite regulation. An imbalanced diet can disrupt their production and lead to overeating. The alkaline diet's emphasis on whole, nutrient-dense foods may promote satiety and better appetite control, indirectly influencing these hormones.

Estrogen

Excess body fat can lead to increased estrogen levels, potentially contributing to hormonal imbalances.

The alkaline diet, which tends to be lower in calorie-dense and processed foods, may support weight management, which can help maintain healthy estrogen levels.

Thyroid Hormones

The alkaline diet encourages the consumption of iodine-rich foods, such as seaweed and sea vegetables, which are essential for proper thyroid function. A well-functioning thyroid gland is crucial for maintaining hormone balance in the body.

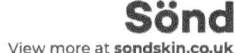

Sex hormones

The alkaline diet's focus on plant-based foods, especially cruciferous vegetables like broccoli and kale, may support liver detoxification. This can aid in the clearance of excess hormones, potentially benefiting sex hormone balance.

Serotonin

A balanced diet rich in vitamins and minerals is crucial for supporting neurotransmitter function, including serotonin production. The alkaline diet's emphasis on nutrient-dense foods may indirectly contribute to improved mood and well-being.

It's important to note that while the alkaline diet may have some potential benefits for hormone balance, hormones are highly complex and influenced by various factors beyond diet alone. Individual responses to dietary changes can vary, and the overall impact of the alkaline diet on hormone balance may differ from person to person.

Are you chewing your food correctly?

Eating food is an everyday occurrence, and although we might give a lot of consideration to what we're eating, especially since we decided to embark on a mostly alkaline diet, we might not give as much consideration to how we eat. This means that we're probably not eating mindfully enough in order to chew our food properly.

Chewing is an important part of the digestive process. Proper chewing involves chewing our food slowly and for longer, keeping it in our mouths for as long as possible with more mindful chews. The benefits of proper chewing include better digestion, more nutrient absorption, less bloating, and lower calorie consumption.

Digestion

Our digestive tract starts in our mouth, then extends through the oesophagus, stomach, small intestine, and large intestine, and then ends at our anus.

Throughout the entire journey, our food undergoes processes that involve digestion, assimilation (the removal of nutrients into the bloodstream), and the absorption of water before being turned into waste.

It's a complex system that needs looking after, with mindful, slow bites of food.

Are you chewing properly?

Most of us fail to chew our food enough. Instead, we take a bite, chew, and swallow, all within seconds.

We need to chew so that we don't choke on large pieces of food passing from our mouths down into our stomachs. But more than that, we need to chew our food in order to start the process of digestion in two ways: mechanical digestion from the act of chewing and chemical digestion as food mixes with the saliva contained within the oral fluid in our mouths.

Mechanical digestion

Mechanical digestion begins to break down the food in our mouths so that we can swallow it and so that it's easier for the rest of the digestive tract to physically break down the food and extract nutrients from it.

Chemical digestion

Chemical digestion starts in the mouth due to the presence of the enzyme amylase in saliva, which breaks down carbohydrates into their constituent parts, sugars.

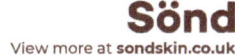

View more at sondskin.co.uk

In fact, most of the digestion of carbohydrates happens in the mouth rather than the stomach.

If we don't keep our food in our mouth long enough, partially digested carbohydrates will pass into the stomach, where the stomach will have to work harder to digest them, potentially leading to bloating, stomach pains, and constipation. Unlike carbohydrates, proteins and fats are broken down in the stomach due to the presence of two different digestive enzymes, protease and lipase, that break down proteins and fats, respectively.

Are you "Good and Hungry"?

In the early 1900s, a food writer and academic named Horace Fletcher began to lecture on the power of mastication—mastication being the scientific word for chewing.

He earned himself the nickname *The Great Masticator* due to his argument that food should be masticated thoroughly "until liquefied" before swallowing. "Nature will castigate those who don't masticate," he was very fond of saying.

His argument at the time was that his method of chewing food (and even liquids in order to mix them with saliva) "increased the amount of strength" someone could have, while at the same time decreasing the amount of food they would eat.

Fletcher advocated the following:

- Eat only when you have a good appetite or when you're "good and hungry."
- Chew your food to a pulp before swallowing.
- Do not drink in gulps; instead, sip liquids.

This then became known as the Theory of Fletcherism, which highlighted the importance of chewing.

It also introduced the concept of emotional eating—that is, the importance of only eating when we're hungry rather than grazing and snacking when we're not feeling hungry and when we're instead feeling emotional (either in a happy or a sad sense). Fletcher, in fact, advised against eating when we're angry, stressed, upset, or worried.

I advocate for much of this theory, especially eating mindfully when you're hungry and purposefully chewing your food. When it comes to drinking, I agree on sipping rather than gulping, but I don't advise drinking water or any other liquid while eating.

Doing so will dilute the saliva, which isn't helpful for digestion. Instead, drink water before and after each meal.

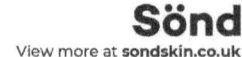

The benefits of chewing more slowly

Our digestive processes can be helped by chewing our food carefully and mindfully.

We will then absorb nutrients more efficiently, not least because carbohydrates begin their digestion journey in the mouth (and the longer our food stays in the mouth, the more digestion occurs). But also because the process of chewing stimulates saliva production as well as activating digestive processes in the stomach, pancreas, and small intestine.

If these organs don't receive these messages because we swallow our food too quickly, they're ill-prepared, and food will move more sluggishly. This means less efficient nutrient absorption.

When our stomach, pancreas, and small intestines are also ready and prepared for food to digest, it makes the process smoother, meaning less indigestion, bloating, gas, pain, nausea, reflux, headaches, and constipation.

We also tend to consume fewer calories if we eat more slowly. Studies show that if we slow down our chewing, we reduce the amount of food we need to eat because our satiety-triggering hormone, leptin (which tells us that we're full), is released sooner.

It's generally accepted that "slow chewing" means chewing each mouthful between 32 and 52 times.

How to chew more

The aim is to increase the number of times you chew from your normal, 'baseline' number. Start off mindfully, as the practice of mindful eating encourages us to slow down. This means avoiding all distractions when eating, including the TV, talking, reading, and scrolling on our phones. Concentrate fully on the food you're eating, including its appearance, smell, mouthfeel, texture, and taste.

It's also beneficial to take small mouthfuls, so avoid overloading your cutlery or taking bites that completely fill your mouth. Chew with your mouth closed, using your tongue to move the food from one side of your mouth to the other. Put down your cutlery between mouthfuls too, rather than loading up your fork or spoon ready for the next mouthful while you're still eating your previous one. This will encourage slow, mindful eating. Count your chews, and try to gradually increase them so that it becomes your new normal.

You'll soon be noticing the difference in your digestion, with fewer digestive complaints and possibly even weight loss.

Actions

- Eat mindfully and focus on the food—how it looks, smells, and tastes.
- Take smaller mouthfuls when eating.
- Chew your food until it is fully liquid.

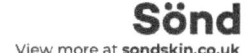

What our stool reveals about our health

In the realm of health discussions, few topics are as avoided as the state of our bowel movements.

Yet, the truth is, our stool can reveal a wealth of information about our overall health and well-being. Understanding the messages hidden in our bathroom habits can empower us to make informed decisions about our diet, lifestyle, and potential health concerns.

Let's embark on a journey to unveil the mysteries behind our stool and discover the valuable insights it offers.

The perfect number: unravelling the frequency

Bowel movements are as individual as we are, but there is a golden rule: three is the magic number. Whether it's three times a day or three times a week, regularity is key.

Straying from this pattern and experiencing infrequent bowel movements might indicate constipation, potentially leading to complications like haemorrhoids.

Embracing this understanding allows us to better gauge our digestive health and make necessary adjustments.

Influences of diet and timing

The foods we eat and the timing of our meals significantly impact our bowel movements. Stimulant-rich beverages like coffee and certain carbonated drinks can speed up the digestive process, leading to more frequent trips to the bathroom. On the contrary, a diet lacking in fibre and water intake can result in infrequent bowel movements. Recognising these important connections empowers us to make mindful dietary choices to support our digestive well-being.

How we go and the time we take

Beyond frequency, how we go and the time spent on the toilet can provide valuable insights. Prolonged periods spent straining on the toilet might indicate constipation or a possible blockage. Frequent urges to pass stool shortly after meals may signify a need for more fibre-rich foods and a reduction in stimulating agents.

Understanding these patterns equips us to optimise our daily routines for better digestive health.

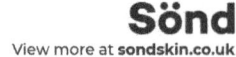

View more at sondskin.co.uk

The Bristol Stool Scale

The Bristol Stool Scale serves as an essential tool for assessing the appearance of our stool. Ranging from hard, separate lumps (Type 1) to entirely liquid with no solid parts (Type 7), it offers a visual representation of stool consistency. The ideal stool falls within Type 4: smooth, sausage-shaped, and easily passed, with a healthy dark brown colour. Observing the scale helps us identify potential issues and maintain digestive balance.

Form, colour, and odour

In addition to consistency, paying attention to stool colour is vital. A very pale or white stool might indicate a blocked bile duct, necessitating medical attention. On the other hand, yellowish stools often correlate with diarrhoea, signalling a rapid passage of food through the digestive system. While we might be hesitant to address the topic of odour, its presence can also provide clues about our diet and gut health.

Floating or sinking

Although not commonly discussed, whether our stool floats or sinks holds significance. Floating stools could result from excessive fibre intake, leading to increased gas production. Conversely, sinking stools are generally considered healthy. Persistent floating stools might indicate malabsorption issues, warranting further investigation and professional consultation.

Our stool is an essential communicator, offering valuable insights into our digestive health and overall well-being. Embracing open conversations about this topic enables us to take proactive steps towards maintaining a healthy gut. By understanding the messages our stool conveys, we can make informed choices about our diet, lifestyle, and potential health concerns. Together, let's empower ourselves with this newfound knowledge and embrace the significance of what our stool reveals about our health.

Actions

- Become conscious of how often and when you go to the toilet.
- If you notice any of the following, we recommend seeing a nutritionist:
    - Floating stools
    - Very light stools
    - Diarrhoea

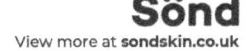

Empowering heavy metal detoxification

In our fast-paced modern world, heavy metal exposure has become a growing concern for our health.

Toxic elements like lead, mercury, cadmium, and arsenic lurk in our environment, posing serious risks to our well-being. Their accumulation in our bodies can lead to a range of health issues, from neurological disorders to kidney damage.

In this section, we will explore the dangers of heavy metal exposure and the pivotal role of an alkaline lifestyle in reducing their levels in our bodies.

Heavy metals, while naturally occurring, have reached alarming levels in the environment due to industrial activities, pollution, and contaminated food and water sources.

These toxic elements find their way into our bodies through various sources, such as polluted water, certain seafood, dental fillings, and even household products.

Their presence disrupts essential biochemical processes and can lead to serious health consequences.

Heavy metals wreak havoc on our health, affecting various bodily systems.

Neurological disorders

Mercury and lead can damage nerve cells, resulting in cognitive decline and neurological disorders.

Cardiovascular issues

Elevated levels of heavy metals contribute to high blood pressure and heart disease.

Kidney damage

Heavy metals impair kidney function, leading to kidney damage and impaired filtration.

Reproductive health

Heavy metal exposure can negatively impact fertility and prenatal development.

Weakened immune system

Heavy metals compromise the immune system's ability to fight off infections.

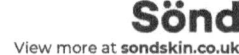

Reducing heavy metal accumulation

Embracing an alkaline lifestyle can significantly aid in reducing heavy metal accumulation in the body.

- An alkaline diet, rich in vegetables and plant based proteins, supports the body's natural detoxification processes, aiding in heavy metal elimination.
- Alkaline foods help maintain the body's pH balance, reducing heavy metal absorption.
- Drinking alkaline water supports efficient toxin removal, including heavy metals.
- An alkaline-rich diet supplies the body with ample antioxidants, neutralising free radicals induced by heavy metals.
- A balanced alkaline lifestyle fortifies the immune system, aiding in heavy metal resistance.

By recognising the dangers of heavy metal exposure and adopting an alkaline lifestyle, we can empower our bodies to reduce heavy metal toxicity effectively.

A diet focused on alkaline foods, regular hydration with alkaline water, and embracing other elements of an alkaline lifestyle provide essential tools for heavy metal detoxification.

Through this proactive approach, we can pave the way for a healthier and more vibrant life, free from the burdens of heavy metal toxicity. Remember, small lifestyle changes can have a significant impact on our well-being and overall health.

Deodorants and antiperspirants

When it comes to personal hygiene, deodorants and antiperspirants have become staples in our daily routines.

The desire to stay fresh and odour-free has led many to rely on these products to combat sweat and prevent unpleasant smells. However, recent concerns have arisen about the potential health risks associated with using antiperspirants containing aluminium compounds.

As we delve into the importance of an alkaline lifestyle, it becomes clear that opting for natural alternatives to these conventional products aligns with our pursuit of improved overall well-being.

Aluminium

Traditional antiperspirants contain aluminium-based compounds, such as aluminium chloride or aluminium zirconium, which temporarily block sweat glands, reducing perspiration. However, these compounds have sparked health concerns due to their absorption into the skin and accumulation in the body over time.

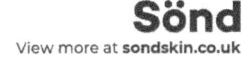

Studies have raised questions about a possible link between aluminium exposure and an increased risk of breast cancer and Alzheimer's disease.

While research is ongoing, the idea of introducing toxins directly into our bodies raises concerns among health conscious individuals.

Shifting towards an alkaline lifestyle involves reevaluating the products we use daily, including our personal care items. By opting for natural deodorants free from harmful chemicals, we not only eliminate the potential health risks associated with antiperspirants but also contribute to a healthier, more balanced body.

An alkaline lifestyle revolves around maintaining a slightly alkaline pH level in the body.

Natural deodorants, typically formulated with gentle, pH-balancing ingredients like baking soda and essential oils, help keep body odour at bay without disrupting the body's pH equilibrium.

Conventional antiperspirants often contain not just aluminium compounds but also parabens, phthalates, and artificial fragrances. By choosing natural deodorants, we avoid exposing our bodies to these potentially harmful substances, promoting a cleaner, toxin free lifestyle.

Sweating is a natural process through which our bodies release toxins.

Traditional antiperspirants hinder this detoxification process, trapping sweat and preventing the elimination of waste. Natural deodorants allow the body to perspire freely, supporting its innate detoxification mechanisms.

Contrary to popular belief, natural deodorants can provide effective odour control. Essential oils, such as lavender, tea tree, and eucalyptus, offer natural antibacterial properties, keeping bacteria at bay and leaving us feeling fresh throughout the day.

Many natural deodorants come in eco friendly packaging and are cruelty free, making them a sustainable choice for both personal and environmental health.

As we embrace the alkaline lifestyle, we acknowledge the significance of adopting natural alternatives that promote a healthier, more balanced life.

Eliminating antiperspirants with aluminium compounds and choosing natural deodorants aligns with our commitment to reducing toxic exposure and supporting our body's natural processes. By making this simple yet impactful shift in our daily routine, we take a step towards overall well-being and a greener, more sustainable world.

So, let us confidently embark on this journey of natural self-care, knowing that our commitment to better health extends beyond ourselves and reaches the world around us.

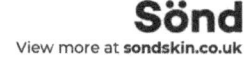

Understanding Ingredients

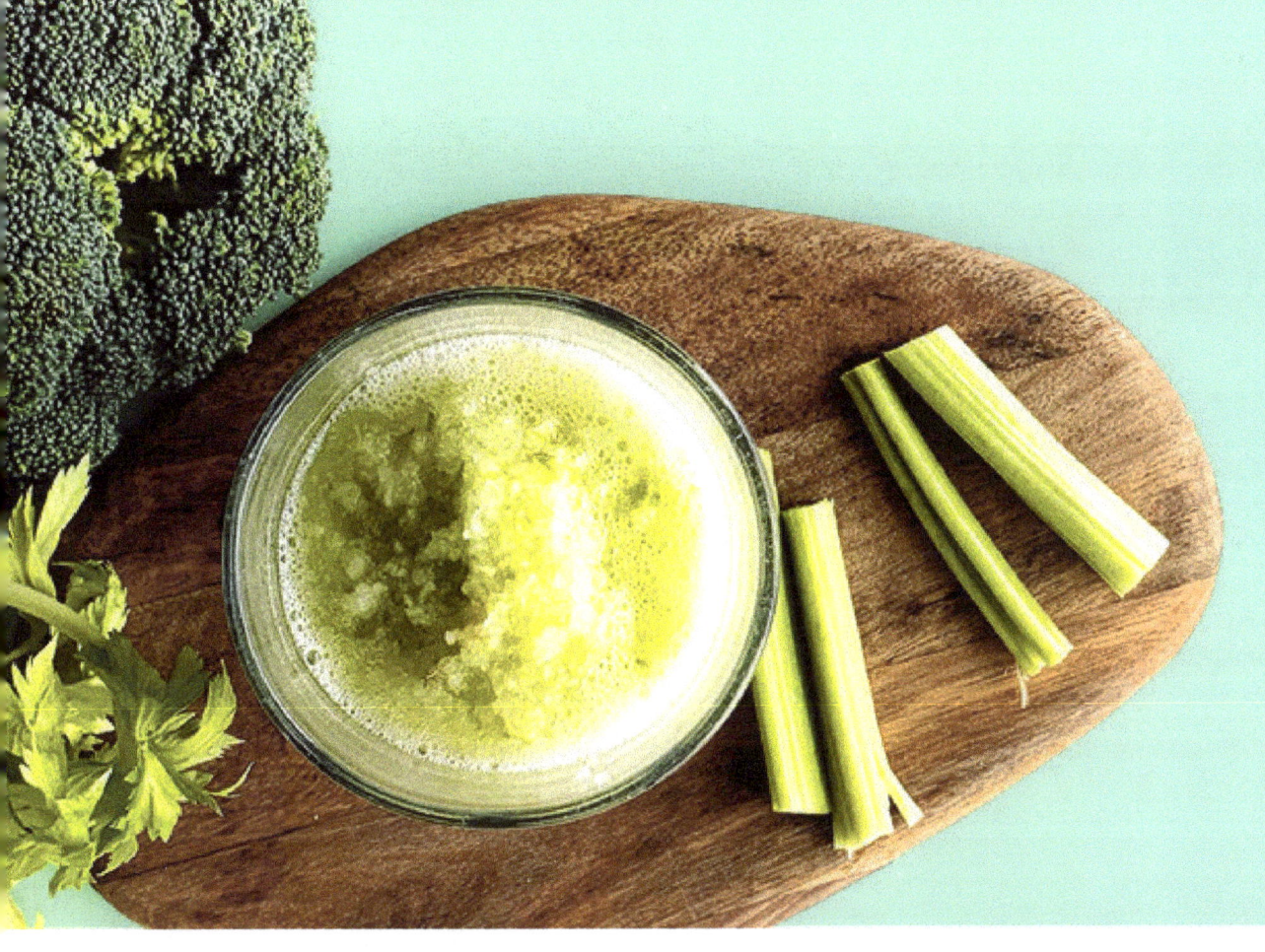

Going green...with your diet

If I asked you how green you were, what would you say?

Like many, you might tell me about your recycling habits or how you visit refill stores to minimise your single-use plastic and always carry a reusable water bottle. All of these are very virtuous habits, but I'm actually asking about your diet. How green is your diet, literally? How many green vegetables do you eat a day?

My advice is to consume five portions of vegetables a day, but I advocate that as a minimum and for green vegetables to feature heavily in our daily diets.

In 2019, the *State of the Nation: Dietary Trends in the UK 20 Years On*, a report by The Health and Food Supplements Information Service (HSIS), found that just 31% of UK adults aged between 19 and 64 years old are reaching the five-a-day target. In the same year, a study published by the American Society for Nutrition concluded that "inadequate fruit and vegetable consumption may account for millions of deaths from heart disease and strokes each year."

The study estimated that around 1 in 12 cardiovascular deaths could be attributed to not eating enough vegetables. Which is pretty shocking when eating vegetables is so enjoyable!

Green, leafy vegetables in particular are packed with valuable nutrients, and most are considered alkaline rather than acid-forming. (See my Alphabet of Alkaline Foods in the previous chapter for a comprehensive list.)

Eating a diet rich in greens means consuming a wide variety of vitamins and minerals that are required for good health. For example, one of the most nutrient-dense vegetables is kale, which provides vitamins A, C, and K, the minerals calcium, potassium, copper, and manganese, plus the antioxidants lutein and beta-carotene. Green, leafy vegetables are also rich in fibre, which promotes good gut health.

Eating greens on a daily basis helps with weight management, protects against lifestyle diseases such as type 2 diabetes and heart disease, promotes clear skin, and supports good emotional wellbeing. What's more, adding more greens to our diet is really simple.

Just by following one of my upcoming five tips for adding more greens to your diet, you'll be topping up on delicious, nutrient-packed, low-calorie foods that support your physical and mental health.

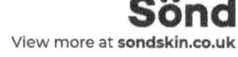

Making a conscious effort to eat more greens will soon become a habit, and good habits such as this help to kickstart good habits elsewhere, making an alkaline lifestyle feel so much easier to adopt.

Creating good habits helps to motivate and empower us, meaning that we'll be more likely to make other healthy choices and form other healthy habits, and it's this philosophy—small steps towards big change—that essentially underpins my alkaline-based approach to natural wellbeing.

5 simple tips to increase your intake of greens

Here are my five tips for increasing your intake of greens, and they're all relatively simple to incorporate into your life.

Start with one and build up to as many as you like; that way, you won't become overwhelmed with too many "rules" surrounding your food, and you'll be more likely to stick to them.

Before you know it, it'll be second nature to eat lots of delicious greens every single day!

One

Start each day with green juice. During your detox week, you will get used to drinking red and green juices throughout the day, so try to carry on this habit with at least one green juice (feel free to add a red one in too) per day. Starting the morning with green juice after detoxifying lemon tea helps set a healthy trend.

My green juice recipe is packed with green leaves and a zingy, zesty, wake-me-up kick from the ginger and lemon. It's also five vegetable portions in one hit before you've even started work, so who knows how many more you'll add during the day?

Two

Add a green salad to your midday and evening meals. A green salad couldn't be easier to prepare; it's simply two handfuls of salad leaves, a squeeze of lemon, and a drizzle of extra virgin olive oil. If you like, add some fresh basil or coriander. Place it all in a bowl and serve it with whatever you have for lunch and dinner.

Three

When you're making soups, stews, or curries, add a generous handful of spinach leaves to the pot, right at the very end after you've removed it from the heat. Spinach quickly wilts in hot food or steam and adds a delicious dose of greens to any dish.

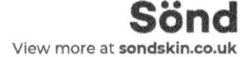

Four

Other green alkaline vegetables can be added to freshly prepared soups and stews, but if you're eating a raw meal, you don't have to miss out on nutrient packed kale, Brussels sprouts, and broccoli that can all be eaten raw. Kale is delicious mixed with a little extra virgin olive oil and massaged to break down some of the fibre content, and broccoli and brussel sprouts can be grated over the top of dishes in the same way that Parmesan cheese would be in an Italian restaurant.

Five

If you fancy eating pasta, I'd always recommend opting for a gluten free version and never eating white pasta. But one step better is to make courgette spaghetti using a spiraliser. Sometimes called zoodles (zucchini noodles), courgette spaghetti can be eaten raw or blanched in hot water for a minute. If you do opt for gluten free pasta, spinach, kale, collard greens, beetroot, and dandelion leaves can all be roughly chopped and added to the pasta water towards the end of the cooking time for added greens.

Never underestimate the power of eating green, leafy vegetables, and never underestimate how easy it is to add more greens to your diet.

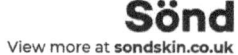

Demystifying gluten

Gluten is found in many different foods, the most obvious being foods made from wheat, such as bread and pasta. But gluten can also be found in ready made soups and sauces, and even some beer and nutritional supplements.

There's a lot of talk around gluten, all of which ultimately elaborates on the question of whether we should be eating it or not?

If you have a gluten allergy or the autoimmune condition coeliac disease, then your medical doctors would've told you to completely eliminate it from your diet. If you don't have a gluten allergy, but consuming gluten causes you to experience abdominal discomfort and headaches, then you may have a gluten intolerance. (Those with a gluten intolerance need to avoid it completely for three months before slowly reintroducing it a little bit at a time, under the guidance of a nutritionist.)

During your seven day detox, all foods that contain gluten are to be avoided. After your detox, you may introduce gluten into your diet, but I advise keeping it to a minimum by choosing gluten free bread and pasta and avoiding all processed foods.

If you do choose to eat gluten containing foods, make sure you choose whole grain versions that have been minimally processed.

What is gluten?

Despite most commonly being found in carbohydrate-based foods, gluten is actually a protein. It occurs naturally in wheat as well as other grains such as rye and barley. Some oat products also contain gluten, but oats themselves are naturally gluten free. Oat products can become contaminated with gluten as a consequence of being processed alongside other gluten containing grains.

Foods such as shop bought soups and sauces contain concentrated gluten as an added ingredient after the gluten has been extracted from wheat, rye, or barley. In these processed foods, gluten doesn't much resemble the naturally occurring gluten found in wheat and is used as a thickening agent, adding texture and binding food together.

When we consume gluten, the gut uses the enzyme protease to break down the protein into amino acids ready for digestion. However, protease cannot completely break down gluten.

As a result, some undigested gluten then travels to the small intestine, where it can begin to cause unpleasant symptoms including abdominal pain and bloating, nausea, diarrhoea, headaches, and skin rashes.

If you have coeliac disease, this partially digested gluten then causes an autoimmune response and, over time, can cause severe damage to the lining of the small intestine.

Leaky gut

Some people may experience these symptoms even if they don't have coeliac disease, because they may have a leaky gut. A leaky gut is difficult to diagnose and is a condition that allows undigested gluten to leak into the bloodstream, causing inflammation that can lead to the symptoms mentioned above.

Those with a sensitive gut may also experience these symptoms as a result of undigested, fermenting carbohydrates called FODMAPS (fermentable oligosaccharides, disaccharides, monosaccharides, and polyols) passing through the small intestine, not just gluten.

Either way, my advice will always be to minimise the level of gluten in your diet and to completely eliminate it from your diet during detox week (and beyond if you have coeliac disease).

Healthy microbiome

There is evidence that consuming a low gluten diet supports a healthy microbiome, the collection of viruses, bacteria, and other microorganisms that reside in our gut.

A healthy microbiome is linked to better gut health, and emerging evidence suggests that it also supports other areas of health, such as our immune health and mental wellbeing.

A low gluten diet can also reduce gut problems such as pain and bloating and can even promote weight loss.

It's been suggested that eliminating gluten could result in a deficiency of certain micronutrients, including the B vitamins. But if you consume plenty of leafy greens, legumes, and seeds as part of your alkaline lifestyle, you'll still be consuming a sufficient level of B vitamins.

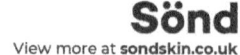

Everything you need to know about sugar

Refined sugar really isn't welcome in any diet, especially not a healthy, wholesome diet, and least of all on the alkaline lifestyle diet.

Refined sugar, or white, granulated table sugar, otherwise known as sucrose, is found in all manner of foods, from sweets and chocolate to cakes, biscuits, and pastries, as well as fizzy drinks and artificial fruit drinks. It's even found in some savoury foods, such as shop bought soups, sauces, and condiments.

Sugar promotes inflammation

Sugar is an acid-forming food that promotes inflammation, which, if left unchecked, can become chronic and lead to chronic inflammatory diseases such as obesity, type 2 diabetes, and heart disease.

Eating a diet high in sugary foods (including processed carbohydrates such as white bread, pasta, and rice that are quickly turned into sugar called glucose during digestion) is a surefire journey to inflammation and disease. It can undo all the good work you're doing by eating alkaline, anti-inflammatory foods. So it's best to keep sweet treats to a minimum.

Look out for sugar listed in the ingredients of shop bought foods; the higher it appears in the ingredients list, the more sugar the product will contain.

Food manufacturers are crafty too and will sneak sugar into their recipes and call it something different.

If you're planning to eat pre-packaged food, look out for the following on the ingredient list, as they're refined sugars in disguise:

- High-fructose corn syrup
- Corn syrup
- Invert sugar
- Barley malt syrup
- Malt syrup
- Cane juice/sugar
- Palm sugar
- Raw sugar

Pretty much anything that contains the words sugar or syrup is added sugar.

Carbohydrates and sugar

The body requires a certain amount of sugar in order to function, and its preferred source is glucose (the term "blood sugar level" refers to the level of glucose circulating in the blood).

Certain vegetables and the carbohydrates in bread and pasta provide the glucose that the body needs. Starchy and unrefined carbohydrates such as those found in vegetables, brown bread, and pasta are broken down into glucose by the body slowly and sustainably, providing a steady, slow-release form of energy.

On the other hand, refined carbohydrates (white bread and pasta) are broken down quickly, flooding the blood with glucose and giving us immediate energy. But this high is quickly followed by a low, and we end up feeling sluggish and lethargic, craving another high and more sugar.

The same happens when we eat sweets, cakes, and biscuits. Eating refined carbohydrates and sugary foods puts us in a vicious downward spiral.

Fructose and the liver

Fruit is sweet because it contains a type of sugar called fructose. Throughout this book, you'll have noticed that during detox week and beyond, I place most of my emphasis on vegetables, less so on fruit.

This is primarily because most vegetables are alkaline (see my Alphabet of Alkaline Foods) and not many fruits are. But it's also because of fructose that is in fruit.

Fruit isn't inherently bad; it's packed with vitamins and antioxidants, but we should concentrate on a higher intake of vegetables over fruit. There are, however, many problems associated with consuming high levels of fruit sugar. Fruit sugar in the form of high fructose corn syrup, which we can see from our list above, is a refined sugar that's used to sweeten processed foods.

Fruit should only be eaten because by making juice, you remove the fibers,

leaving only fructose that goes directly to the liver, putting the liver under stress.

Glucose is metabolised by every cell in the body for energy. Fructose is metabolised almost entirely by the liver.

When we consume high fructose corn syrup, the liver is placed under immense stress to metabolise this sugar, preventing it from getting on with its other important functions. The liver is responsible for processing digested food, controlling fat and glucose levels in the blood, filtering pathogens from the blood, neutralising toxins, manufacturing bile, storing iron and vitamins, regulating hormones, and manufacturing enzymes.

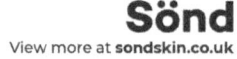

The liver has an exhausting job, and if we flood it with too much fructose, especially high fructose corn syrup, it will store it as fat. This can then lead to weight gain, especially due to an increase in dangerous visceral fat (the fat that surrounds the organs and is notoriously difficult to shift), fatty liver disease, insulin resistance (which can lead to prediabetes and type 2 diabetes), and chronic inflammation.

What's more, consuming lots of high fructose corn syrup can interfere with the hunger hormones ghrelin and leptin. Ghrelin is released when our stomach is empty and signals to us that we're hungry, effectively increasing our appetite. Leptin is the opposite of ghrelin and is released when we're full, signalling to us that we need to stop eating.

So it's clear that if these are interfered with, it could lead to confusion over our hunger cues, never feeling full, and potential weight gain.

Also, when fructose is metabolised, two types of saturated fat are produced: stearic acid and palmitic acid, and these in turn can increase levels of so-called bad cholesterol, LDL, or low-density lipoprotein. High LDL levels can then lead to an increased risk of heart disease.

Choose from this list if you'd like to add occasional sweetness to your diet. I've listed them in order of preference according to the percentage of fructose, from 'best' to 'worst'.

Finally, fructose causes more extreme blood sugar spikes than glucose, resulting in hastily raised insulin levels, which trigger the adrenal glands to produce more of the stress hormone cortisol, leading to adrenal fatigue, which can cause body aches, lethargy, and dizziness.

Exhausting, for sure.

Alternatives to sugar

So it's clear that we need to avoid foods with added sugars such as sucrose and fructose syrups as much as possible. But if we fancy sweetening food occasionally, then we do have options.

These alternatives are still sugar and should be used sparingly (and definitely not daily), but they cause less severe blood sugar spikes and can help to gradually wean us off sugar for good.

Stevia

Stevia, a relative newcomer, Stevia is a fructose-free, zero-calorie sweetener made from plants. It's 300 times sweeter than sucrose and therefore should be used in tiny amounts.

Use stevia in baking to sweeten hot drinks, and sprinkle it over dishes you want to add a little sweetness to. Take care not to use too much, as it can have a bitter aftertaste.

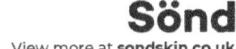

Brown rice syrup

Made using fermented brown rice, this syrup is also free from fructose and is similar in texture and taste to maple syrup. Use it in baking and as a drizzle or topping.

Monk fruit extract

Monk fruit extract is similar to stevia in that it's derived from plants, is hundreds of times sweeter than sucrose, contains zero calories, and is fructose-free. Use it in place of table sugar.

Yacon syrup

Rich in inulin, a prebiotic fibre that feeds the good bacteria and viruses in the gut, yacon syrup contains roughly 30% fructose. It has a slightly 'overcooked' taste, so it is best used in baking where the taste can be disguised.

Honey

High quality unprocessed honey, such as Manuka or Jarrah honey, is prized for its medicinal qualities, such as its antimicrobial and antioxidant properties. But it's worth keeping in mind that honey is 40–50% fructose, meaning that in terms of the liver, it doesn't fare much better than high fructose corn syrup.

Use in smoothies and over cereals. Honey is an animal product, so if you're consuming a plant based diet, avoid using honey.

Coconut syrup

Despite its name, coconut syrup (also available as coconut sugar) doesn't taste anything like coconuts. It's 40% fructose, made from the nectar of the flowering coconut tree, and is best used in baking.

Molasses

Often made from sugar cane or sugar beet juice, molasses is around 40–50% fructose. A dark, treacle-like liquid, molasses, can be used in baking.

Maple syrup

Made from boiling down the sap of the maple tree until a syrup is formed, maple syrup is around 35–40% fructose.

It can be used in baking and as a drizzle or topping.

Agave syrup

Made from the same Mexican plant that's used to make tequila, agave syrup can come in two forms: light and dark. Light agave syrup is filtered and has a lighter taste. I really wouldn't recommend using either agave syrup, as it can contain up to 80–90% fructose!

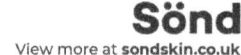

Xylitol

Xylitol is 100% fructose free, but it's also extremely refined, and as such I'd therefore suggest avoiding this sugar alternative altogether.

Actions

- Keep your sugar intake to a minimum as much as possible.
- Avoid refined carbohydrates like white bread.
- Try to consume no more than one portion of fruit per day.

Dairy vs non-dairy – making the switch

Humans are the only species on Earth to drink the milk of another species.

No other species does this—a puppy wouldn't naturally suckle from a mother cat, just as a baby giraffe in the wild wouldn't drink from the teat of a wild antelope mother.

Yet for hundreds of years, it's been accepted practice to feed human babies and children the milk of a mother cow, and for this to continue happening as we grow into adults (unlike most animals who stop drinking milk at a young age).

Cow's milk and other dairy products, such as cheese and yoghurt, contain micronutrients and protein that help youngsters grow and develop normally and that nourish fully grown adults. But there's also a well-known saying: *"If you've got milk, you've likely got a host of health problems awaiting you too."*

Drinking cow's milk and eating dairy made using cow's milk (or any other animal-based milk) means consuming acid-forming food and drink.

Therefore, I've eliminated all dairy from my seven day detox and advise that it's only consumed minimally as part of your 80:20 alkaline diet.

Dairy is acid forming

When we consume animal products such as meat and dairy, our body produces acid. Calcium, an important mineral for the health and strength of our bones and teeth, as well as for muscle function, is an effective acid neutraliser. Therefore, when we consume dairy, calcium from the dairy product as well as calcium from our bones is used to neutralise the resulting acid, taking it away from its important job of keeping the bones strong. Which is ironic, given that the dairy industry has for decades used clever marketing tactics to convince us that drinking milk is the "best" way to keep our bones healthy. In fact, studies show that those who consume the highest amount of dairy products actually also experience higher rates of bone fractures.

A study published in the "British Medical Journal" in 2014, titled "Milk intake and risk of mortality and fractures in women and men: cohort studies," conducted by Michaelsson et al., suggested that high milk intake in both women and men was associated with higher mortality and fracture risk.

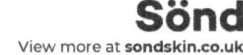

View more at sondskin.co.uk

Hormones

Dairy milk naturally contains animal hormones, including the two female sex hormones, oestrogen and progesterone. Studies suggest a possible link between consuming cow hormones and human cancers of the breast, womb, and prostate. Oestrogen is a fat soluble hormone and is therefore found in higher concentrations in full fat dairy milk than semi skimmed or skimmed milk.

In some countries, dairy herds are also fed artificial growth hormones that can be present in their milk. The use of growth hormones in dairy herds is banned in the UK.

Antibiotics

In addition to hormones, dairy milk often contains traces of antibiotics used to treat a common infection of the udders of dairy cows called mastitis. These antibiotics are problematic when they inevitably enter the human food chain because antibiotic resistance is an increasingly worrying problem.

On an individual level, this means we're unwittingly consuming antibiotics with our milk and that we might need stronger and stronger antibiotics to cure a simple illness such as a bacterial throat infection or urine infection in the future. On a community, national, and global level, antibiotic resistance is worrying on a much larger scale; the antibiotic apocalypse is said to be the next major threat to humankind.

Fats

Full-fat dairy products, especially cheese, contain high levels of saturated fat and cholesterol. Regularly consuming milk and dairy products can therefore lead to weight gain, obesity, high cholesterol, high blood pressure, and heart disease. Adding to the problem is the high level of sodium, or salt, also found in cheese.

Carcinogens

As if all that isn't enough, it's been said (by biochemist T. Colin Campbell) that "casein is the most relevant carcinogen ever found." Casein is the main protein found in milk, and while studies are still looking into this claim, research published in the "British Journal of Cancer" in 2013, and conducted at the University of Illinois indicated that casein intake could potentially influence the proliferation of prostate cancer cells. The study suggested that a diet high in casein might promote prostate tumour growth.

Acne causing

Our skin doesn't escape either, A systematic review and meta-analysis published in the "Journal of the European Academy of Dermatology and Venereology" in 2018 reported a positive association between dairy consumption, particularly skimmed milk, and acne.

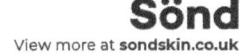

Intolerances and allergies

Lactose intolerance (an intolerance to lactose, the sugar naturally found in dairy milk) is also an increasing problem. It can result in symptoms including headaches, bloating, stomach cramps, nausea, diarrhoea and vomiting.

Worse than this, a milk allergy, that is, a potentially severe allergic reaction to milk, including anaphylaxis, especially in young children, is also a very real problem for many.

Choosing dairy free options

During your seven day detox, all dairy is eliminated, including dairy alternatives such as oat milk. But after your detox, when you're living your alkaline lifestyle, if you like, you can introduce some dairy milk alternatives, as long as you're still within the 80:20 balance.

With vegan and plant based diets becoming more mainstream, food manufacturers, both old and new, are cottoning on, and there are now many plant based alternatives to milk and dairy products.

Dairy free milks made from oats, almonds, peas, hemp, tiger nuts, rice, and coconut are all now freely available.

I recommend almond, oat and coconut as the best for fitting into your alkaline diet. Oat milk is good in coffee if you're drinking it; almond milk is not so good as it often splits (unless it's a barista version). Almond milk goes well with sprouted grains and cereals. Coconut milk has a creamy, distinct, sometimes sweet or overpowering taste and is great for baking, whereas oat milk is pretty much indistinguishable in taste from cow's milk.

Humans have evolved to only truly tolerate the milk of one animal: humans. Human breast milk contains everything a baby needs in order to grow, and the World Health Organisation (WHO) recommends that babies be breastfed until they're two years old for this reason.

Adults wishing to consume milk in keeping with their evolution should therefore arguably only consume plant based milk, so do some experimenting and make the switch as part of your alkaline-based approach to natural wellbeing.

Actions

- Reduce your dairy consumption so that it falls within your 80:20 alkaline/acid diet.
- Start introducing dairy alternatives into your diet.

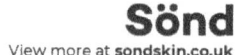

Embracing healthy fats

In the pursuit of a healthy lifestyle, fats have often been perceived as the enemy, leading many to adopt low-fat or fat-free diets. However, not all fats are created equal.

In fact, healthy fats are essential for our overall well-being and play a vital role in maintaining optimal health. This section aims to shed light on the importance of healthy fats and the adverse effects of bad fats on our bodies.

Healthy fats are an essential part of a balanced diet and offer numerous health benefits. Some examples of healthy fats include:

Omega-3s, found in fatty fish, flaxseeds, and walnuts, are renowned for their anti-inflammatory properties, supporting heart health and promoting brain function.

Omega-6s, present in various vegetable oils and nuts, are vital for the body's overall health, but an excessive intake might contribute to inflammation.

Omega-9s, often found in olive oil and avocados, are monounsaturated fats that aid in reducing bad cholesterol levels and promoting heart health, playing a role in a well-rounded healthy diet.

Fats are to be consumed in ratio 2:1:1 for Omega 3, Omega 6 and Omega 9

Foods that contain healthy fats

Incorporating healthy fats into our diet is essential for promoting overall health and well-being. We can do this by choosing sources like:

- Avocados
- Nuts
- Seeds
- Olive oil

Eating healthy fats has multiple health benefits, which are outlined below.

Nutrient absorption

Healthy fats, such as monounsaturated and polyunsaturated fats, are essential for the absorption of fat-soluble vitamins (A, D, E, and K).

These vitamins are crucial for various bodily functions, including immune support, bone health, and vision.

Heart health

Contrary to popular belief, certain fats are heart-protective. Omega-3 fatty acids, found in fatty fish like salmon and flaxseeds, have been shown to reduce inflammation, lower triglyceride levels, and improve heart health.

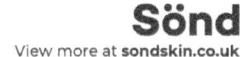

Brain function

The brain is composed of approximately 60% fat, with omega-3s playing a vital role in brain development and cognitive function. Including healthy fats in our diet can boost memory, concentration, and overall brain health.

Hormone regulation

Healthy fats are essential for hormone production and balance. They support the synthesis of sex hormones like oestrogen and testosterone, as well as stress-regulating hormones like cortisol.

Satiety and weight management

Healthy fats contribute to a feeling of fullness and satisfaction after meals, reducing the likelihood of overeating and aiding in weight management.

Fats to avoid

It is crucial to limit the intake of unhealthy fats to safeguard our health and reduce the risk of chronic diseases.

Trans fats

Artificially produced trans fats, often found in processed foods and margarine, have been linked to an increased risk of heart disease, inflammation, and insulin resistance.

It is essential to avoid trans fats in our diet whenever possible.

Saturated fats

While saturated fats are not all bad, excessive consumption of saturated fats, primarily from animal sources like red meat and full-fat dairy, can raise LDL cholesterol levels and increase the risk of heart disease.

Side effects of unhealthy fats:

Eating unhealthy fats can lead to health issues, which I will outline next.

Weight gain and obesity

Diets high in unhealthy fats, especially trans fats and excessive saturated fats, have been associated with weight gain and obesity due to their high caloric content and negative impact on appetite regulation.

Impaired blood vessels

Unhealthy fats can lead to the buildup of plaque in our arteries, reducing blood flow and increasing the risk of hypertension and cardiovascular diseases.

Cognitive decline

Research suggests that diets high in unhealthy fats may contribute to cognitive decline and an increased risk of neurodegenerative diseases like Alzheimer's disease.

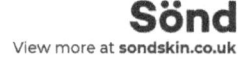

The hidden dangers of low-fat and fat-free foods

In our quest for healthier eating habits, many of us have enthusiastically turned to low-fat or fat-free food options, believing they are the key to a slimmer and more balanced lifestyle.

However, while these products may seem like the perfect solution for cutting down on calories and reducing fat intake, there are hidden dangers that deserve our attention.

Sugar overload

To compensate for the loss of flavour when removing fat, manufacturers often add excessive amounts of sugar to low-fat or fat-free foods. This high sugar content can wreak havoc on our health, leading to weight gain, insulin resistance, and an increased risk of developing chronic diseases like diabetes and heart conditions.

Unhealthy ingredients

In the pursuit of making fat-free products taste appealing, artificial additives, preservatives, and flavour enhancers are commonly used.

These chemicals can have adverse effects on our digestive system and overall well-being.

Unsatisfying and unsustainable

Low-fat and fat-free foods often leave us feeling unsatisfied and hungry shortly after consumption.

This can lead to overeating and an inability to maintain the diet long-term, ultimately sabotaging our efforts to live a healthier lifestyle.

Nutrient depletion

Fat plays a crucial role in the absorption of certain essential vitamins, such as vitamins A, D, E, and K. Consuming fat-free foods can lead to a deficiency in these vital nutrients, negatively impacting our immune system, bone health, and overall vitality.

Impact on hormonal balance

Dietary fat is essential for the production of hormones, including those that regulate our metabolism and promote feelings of satiety.

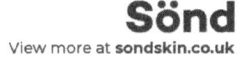
View more at sondskin.co.uk

Restricting fat intake excessively can disrupt hormonal balance and lead to hormonal imbalances.

Effects on mental health

While some observational studies have suggested potential links between dietary fat intake and mental health, the research in this area is complex and ongoing.

However, a study published in 2009 in the "Journal of Affective Disorders" titled "Dietary fat intake and the risk of depression: The SUN (Seguimiento Universidad de Navarra) Project" examined the relationship between different types of dietary fats and the incidence of depression among 12,059 participants in the SUN Project.

This study found that a higher intake of trans fats (unhealthy fats found in processed foods) was associated with a higher risk of depression, while monounsaturated and polyunsaturated fats showed some potential protective effects against depression.

In light of these concerns, it is essential to approach low-fat or fat-free products with caution and scepticism.

Rather than focusing solely on reducing fat intake, we should prioritise consuming a balanced diet rich in whole, natural foods. Incorporating healthy fats from sources like avocados, nuts, seeds, and olive oil can actually benefit our health and contribute to an overall sense of well-being.

Remember, true health comes from making informed and sustainable choices that nourish both our bodies and minds. Let's steer away from the allure of quick-fix diets and embrace a lifestyle that supports long-term health and happiness.

Drinks

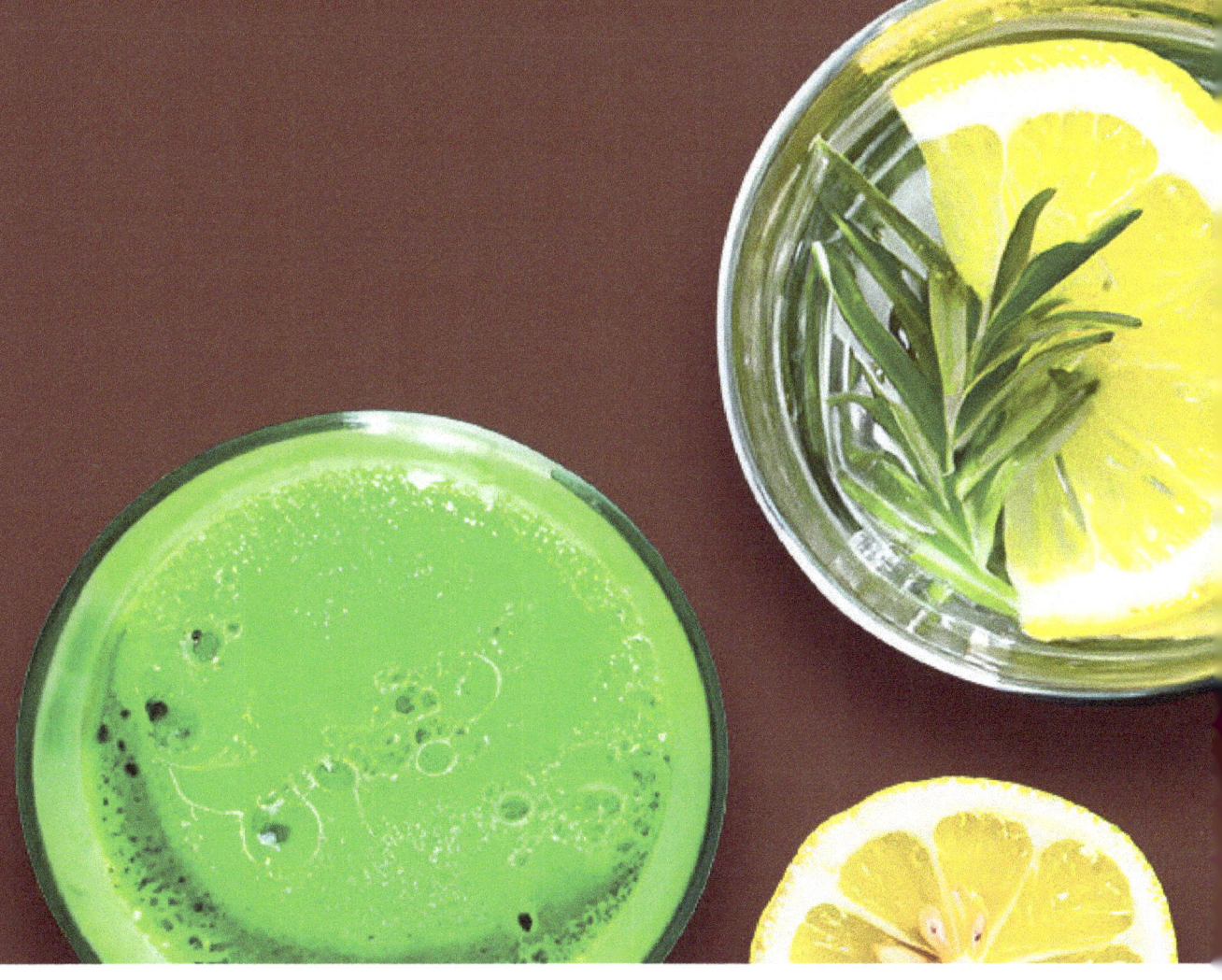

Why water is the key to health

Doctors and health professionals will always tell you to drink more water. This isn't vague, unsubstantiated advice - it really is the key to our health. Without adequate hydration, our body is unable to function properly or achieve optimum wellbeing. Our bodies will store acids, toxins and metabolic waste and in turn, our immune system, internal organs and skin will suffer.

Drinking 2-3 litres of water every single day is essential, and preferably the water we drink is not chemically treated water from the kitchen tap. The best water can be purchased with extra minerals added, and toxins and other harmful substances removed, and there are a few different types:

- Alkaline water—ideal for health, detoxification and longevity
- Mineralised water—essential for optimum hydration
- Cleansing water—helps cells to release toxic waste
- Nourishing water—with a balanced range of essential minerals
- Hydrating water—instantly hydrates at a cellular level
- Energising water—filled with healthy electrolytes for vitality
- Antioxidant water—helps eliminate free radicals
- Excellent quality water—clean and fresh with a good taste

Water is far more than H2O!

The Eastern Perspective

In Eastern philosophy, a very different question is asked of water and has been for hundreds of years. Eastern healers ask, 'What are the properties of water that are needed to support life, vitality and wellbeing?'

The result of this questioning has resulted in the following:

- Toxins, contaminants and chemicals must be filtered out of water
- Water must contain a balanced range of alkaline minerals for absorption by the body
- The chemical structure of water must be hexagonal, with clusters small enough for absorption at a cellular level.

Filtering water is relatively simple, but it's only halfway there. To achieve the full 100% of the Eastern philosophy, we must again ask, 'What are the properties of natural spring water that support health and wellbeing?'

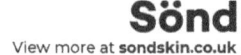
View more at sondskin.co.uk

By asking this question we discover that Mother Nature's water cycle doesn't produce water that is simply H2O. It produces an energised and specifically structured and balanced water that benefits our body and improves our wellbeing. Most importantly, it's in a state that our body can receive and absorb well.

Minerals in water

As it travels through the earth, filtering through natural sand, soil and mineral deposits, water loses toxins and picks up minerals, magnetic energy from Mother Earth and infrared energy from the sun. Its structure also changes and adapts. By the time it bubbles from a spring and flows down a stream, water contains important properties that are essential for our hydration and essential for life. It becomes water that contains the right properties, including a balanced range of minerals, that is readily received and absorbed into the body for optimal cellular hydration.

Electrolytes in water

Potassium, sodium and chloride are key electrolyte minerals, helping to keep the levels of water in the body in balance. The water we choose to drink has to contain a complete and balanced range of alkaline minerals including these three important electrolytes.

An electrolyte is a mineral that dissolves in water and carries an electrical charge (they're also referred to as alkaline minerals and mineral salts). There are many different electrolytes, but the most important ones are:

- Sodium
- Chloride
- Potassium
- Bicarbonate
- Calcium
- Phosphate.

Electrolytes in the body

Our kidneys have specific transporters that regulate the concentration of each of these electrolytes in our blood. Since the body is mostly made up of water (75% of the body and 91% of the brain are made up of water), electrolytes are found everywhere in the body: inside the cells, in the spaces between cells, in the blood, in lymph glands, and everywhere else. When we sweat, we lose fluids and electrolytes.

Sodium has a positive charge, as does potassium, while chloride has a negative charge. Because electrolytes have electrical charges, they can easily move back and forth through the cell membranes. This is important because as they move into a cell, they carry other nutrients in with them, and as they move out, they carry away acidic metabolic waste products and also excess water.

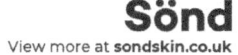

Magnesium is used in nearly every bodily function; it's considered our master mineral! Yet most of us need additional magnesium because we don't consume enough.

Balance

To keep body fluid levels in balance, our cells need to have high levels of potassium inside them and high levels of sodium in the fluids outside them. To maintain balance, sodium and potassium constantly move back and forth through the cell membranes.

Sodium

Sodium easily combines with other elements and is necessary to make hydrochloric acid, the powerful digestive juice inside our stomach that breaks down food to enable it to be digested and absorbed. As the electrolytes are absorbed, water follows. Sodium also minimises urination. When we're drinking good quality water, it will stay in our body longer, giving it more time to become absorbed, which will help us stay in balance and hydrated for longer.

All three electrolytes—sodium, potassium, and chloride—help to keep the amount of water in the body in balance, carry impulses along the nerves, make muscles contract and relax, and keep the body from becoming too acidic or alkaline.

So now we can see the importance of good quality, mineralised water!

Further Benefits of Staying Hydrated

Drinking mineralised water also helps to slow down the natural ageing process as it helps cellular renewal in the skin and helps to protect the skin from the damaging effects of free radicals. What's more, well-hydrated skin is healthy, glowing skin since our skin is the main organ responsible for eliminating toxins through sweat.

Staying well hydrated also helps to clear toxins from the body, which helps to support a good metabolism.

Having a healthy metabolic rate means that we're also more likely to lose weight or maintain a healthy body weight.

Have you ever felt sluggish and lethargic and couldn't put your finger on why? You may have been dehydrated. Dehydration can lead to brain fog, where we struggle to concentrate, our memory becomes clouded, and we find it difficult to make decisions. Therefore, drinking water can help improve our cognitive function. Our energy levels can significantly improve too, since water helps support the energy carrying ability of our cells.

Tap Water vs Bottled vs Alkalising

Tap water contains toxins in the form of heavy metals, chlorine, and fluoride; therefore, I strongly advise that tap water isn't the answer. Bottled water is also not the answer. Surprisingly, it isn't as regulated as tap water, and we could well be drinking water sold to us as a healthy alternative to tap water that contains anything from arsenic and industrial chemicals to toxic bacteria and pharmaceutical (and illegal) drugs. Bottled water is generally contained within plastic too, which contains known endocrine disruptors such as bisphenol A and phthalates linked to fertility problems and birth abnormalities.

Instead, I advise drinking alkaline water that is rich in minerals and ions. There are alkalising water filters available in shops and online.

The impact of our morning coffee fix

Human beings have an insatiable appetite for coffee, and we think nothing of the money we spend on our habit each year. We wake up convinced that in order to function as human beings, we must drink a cup of strong coffee. We then go about our day, passing places where we can feed our habit, able to buy cup after cup from petrol stations, fast food outlets, pop-up coffee stands, and traditional coffee shops. As life becomes busier and more competitive, we need more and more just to get us through the day. We're then so wired at bedtime that it takes us longer to fall asleep. We spend the night tossing and turning, and we wake up tired the next morning, and so the cycle begins again.

Coffee is a drink used to socialise too; we meet friends for coffee, go on coffee dates, and drink coffee with other parents after the school run. But coffee, or rather caffeine, is a drug—one of the most used drugs in the world. We only need to think of the crushing headaches we get if we go a day (or less) without caffeine to know that it's a drug.

The headache is a sign of withdrawal, a sign that our body is getting rid of a toxin. Caffeine is addictive, and it's a toxin that gives us an acute, artificial stimulus. We're then left craving more when the effects wear off, just like having an addiction to any drug would.

Caffeine has various effects on our bodies. It's a stimulant and keeps us alert and energised, both physically and emotionally. But it also stimulates the production of stress hormones, including cortisol and adrenaline, from the adrenal glands. The effects of which are far from stimulating...

A surge in stress hormones

If you've ever had caffeine jitters from too much coffee, then this is due to a surge of stress hormones in your body, and it's not a nice feeling. Stress hormones are normally produced by the body in times of danger, when we need to flick our fight or flight switch to get us to safety. (Be that ancestorially as we escape from a hungry sabre-toothed tiger or in modern times as we wangle our way out of a stress-inducing work presentation.)

We developed these hormonal stress responses to protect and take care of ourselves. But if we stimulate the adrenal glands constantly by regularly drinking coffee throughout the day, we're placing our body under a lot of stress. In effect, we're eliciting the stress response when we don't necessarily need it, and our stress hormones are surging around the body with nothing to do. We're actually compromising the work of the adrenal glands, which can then lead to adrenal fatigue.

Adrenal fatigue

Adrenal fatigue is a medical condition not yet fully recognised by all doctors, and it's therefore difficult to get a diagnosis. It causes fatigue, body weakness, a loss of appetite, unexplained weight loss, muscle and joint pain, and low blood pressure. Regular caffeine consumption can lead to the symptoms of adrenal fatigue, many of which are quite the opposite of what we hoped for from a cup of coffee.

Damage to the gut lining and nutrient deficiencies

When our body metabolises coffee, it leaves behind chemicals called tannins, in particular tannic acid. Tannic acid can damage the mucous membranes, including the lining of the gut, and cause chronic gastritis. Tannins such as tannic acid can also reduce iron absorption from the gut, potentially causing an iron deficiency. If we're low in iron, we'll feel sluggish and fatigued—again, the opposite of what we'd expect from drinking coffee. Excess tannic acid can also cause nausea, especially if we consume coffee on an empty stomach.

Even the "beneficial" laxative effect of coffee isn't as beneficial as we might first think. It's actually a downside of coffee due to the fact that the caffeine puts our body into a state of stress. The stress hormones released from drinking coffee irritate the lining of the gut, gas is formed, and our bowels undergo an unnatural emptying.

Free radical damage

Coffee is acid-forming, which, if not balanced out with a mostly alkaline diet, can lead to inflammation and disease. The essential process of roasting coffee beans before they reach our cups makes the consumption of coffee even more detrimental to our health.

Raw coffee beans contain some level of fat, but raw coffee beans are inedible and cannot be used to make coffee. When these fats are inevitably exposed to the heat of the bean roasting process, they can become damaged or oxidised. Drinking coffee made from unavoidably oxidised beans then introduces free radicals into the body. Free radicals are nasty, unstable molecules of oxygen that cause damage to our DNA and cells and can lead to oxidative stress, chronic inflammation, and disease.

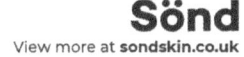

Dull skin, oiliness and acne breakouts

Caffeine is a mild diuretic. A diuretic is something that increases our frequency of urination and can therefore prove to be dehydrating. Dehydration will show in our skin, making it appear dull and sullen. Plus, the cortisol that's released as a consequence of drinking coffee actually triggers the release of sebum, the wax-like substance naturally produced by the skin to protect it and keep it moisturised. Excess sebum will lead to oily skin, blocked pores, spots, and acne breakouts.

Reducing your coffee intake

If you're used to drinking multiple cups of coffee a day, then giving up completely is going to be difficult. Instead, aim to slowly reduce your coffee intake so that you eventually have one cup a day, or even completely eliminate it. During this period, you may experience headaches, constipation, and lethargy for at least a few weeks. It takes around a week for your body to detox from coffee, so the worst symptoms will be felt at the beginning.

Reducing your coffee intake can have significant health benefits, including better sleep, a lower heart rate, and a lower chance of developing dizziness, high blood pressure, and diabetes, making it well worth considering when you're bleary-eyed tomorrow morning!

Actions

- Each week, reduce your coffee intake by one cup per day.
- Once you are down to one cup of coffee per day, try having days where you don't drink coffee and see how you feel.
- If you feel you can, start having coffee as an occasional treat.

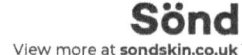

The health impact of tea

Tea, a quintessential beverage, harbours numerous elements that demand attention. Rich in tannins, akin to caffeine, its acidic nature can inflame mucosal linings, potentially leading to sleep disruptions, anxiety, headaches, digestive problems, nausea, and irregular heartbeats—paralleling the effects induced by coffee consumption.

Black tea, being the richest in caffeine content, exacerbates these effects.

Oolong tea contains less caffeine than black tea, while green tea, derived from the Camellia flower, holds the least caffeine content.

Matcha tea

A popular trend is matcha tea, which retains nutrients from the entire tea leaf and boasts higher caffeine and antioxidant content than regular green tea.

Research indicates that matcha contributes to liver protection, heart health, and weight management but still contains caffeine. Despite containing caffeine, Matcha has a lower content than the average cup of coffee. Typically, a cup of matcha contains around 70mg of caffeine, contrasting with the 100-140mg found in a cup of coffee.

However, the unique characteristic of matcha is its ability to sustain alertness for an extended duration in comparison to coffee. While coffee might provide a quick lift for a couple of hours, it often results in a subsequent energy slump, prompting the need for another cup.

Tannin content and iron deficiency

When consuming any form of tea, the body absorbs increased tannin content, a compound that hinders iron absorption in the intestines. Iron deficiency profoundly impacts health, blood circulation, and cognitive functions. Vegetarians relying heavily on plant-based diets face an increased risk of iron deficiency due to the heightened activity of tannins with plant nutrients. Hence, individuals with iron deficiency should consider moderating tea consumption to avoid exacerbating their condition.

The optimal approach is to consume infusions while eliminating any tea.

Infusions are free of caffeine. The name "infusion" refers to the process of steeping plants or fruits in hot water to extract their flavors and nutrients.

Infusions offer several benefits as they are caffeine-free and rich in various nutrients, making them a preferable choice for hydration and health.

Different infusions vary in taste, aroma, and health benefits based on the specific ingredients used.

However, it's essential not to substitute water with tea; hydration should be primarily derived from water intake, even if consuming several cups of tea or infusions.

Alcohol: the impact on health and choosing wisely

Certainly, drinking alcohol can significantly impact our health and well-being. Different types of alcohol, such as spirits, beer, and wine, affect the body in various ways.

In the midst of modern life's stress, alcohol consumption is a common coping mechanism. While the alkaline lifestyle doesn't strictly forbid anything, it emphasizes understanding the consequences of our choices.

Spirits

Due to their high alcohol content, spirits can have detrimental effects on health. The concentrated alcohol levels in spirits contribute to a rapid spike in blood alcohol concentration, which can lead to various health issues.

Excessive consumption of spirits can cause damage to the liver, disrupt sleep patterns, impact mental health, and increase the risk of addiction.

Additionally, the high alcohol content in spirits can irritate the stomach lining and may lead to digestive issues and inflammation.

Cocktails

While enjoyable, contails can have a negative impact on health due to their often high sugar content. Many cocktails contain added sugars, syrups, or sugary mixers to enhance their taste.

Consuming cocktails with high sugar content can contribute to increased caloric intake, potentially leading to weight gain and an elevated risk of conditions like obesity and diabetes.

Additionally, excessive sugar intake from cocktails can cause blood sugar spikes and crashes, leading to energy fluctuations and potential long-term health issues.

Beer

Beer can negatively impact health due to its alcohol content, caloric load, and potential to dehydrate the body. Excessive consumption can contribute to weight gain, worsen health conditions, and compromise overall well-being.

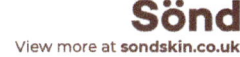

Wine

Savouring a glass of wine can be an experience that transcends taste—it's a journey through culture, tradition, and the art of winemaking. From the lush vineyards to the craftsmanship of fermentation, every sip tells a story that captivates the senses.

White wine often contains high sugar content, while sparkling wine is typically made through a process where a secondary fermentation is induced in the bottle, allowing carbon dioxide to be trapped in the wine, creating characteristic bubbles. The carbonation in sparkling wine can lead to bloating and may cause discomfort in some individuals due to the release of carbon dioxide bubbles.

Acknowledge imperfections and strive for a balanced approach

As a holistic nutritionist, I believe in acknowledging imperfections while striving for a balanced approach to life. While I don't encourage alcohol consumption, I suggest that if one wishes to have a drink occasionally, red wine is a better choice.

Red wine contains Resveratrol, which has numerous potential health benefits such as antioxidant, anti-inflammatory, immunomodulatory, glucose and lipid regulatory, neuroprotective, and cardiovascular protective effects. However, further research is required to substantiate these findings.

When consumed in moderation and complemented by an alkaline lifestyle of nutrient-rich vegetables and foods, an occasional intake of red wine may mitigate potential health risks.

It's crucial to recognize that any alcohol intake can be harmful due to its highly acidic nature and detrimental effects on health.

The OMS (World Health Organization) declared that the appropriate quantity of wine to drink is zero.

It's essential to weigh the potential benefits against the risks and always to remember that moderation and balance are key components in any dietary and lifestyle choices.

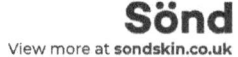

The bitter truth of soft drinks

Soft drinks, often laden with high levels of sugar, artificial sweeteners, and various additives, can have detrimental effects on our health when consumed excessively. Here are some of the negative impacts associated with the regular consumption of soft drinks:

Weight gain and obesity

Soft drinks are notorious for their high sugar content. Regular consumption of sugary beverages can contribute significantly to calorie intake, leading to weight gain and an increased risk of obesity. Excess calories from sugars, especially fructose, are often stored as fat, particularly around the abdomen.

Increased risk of type 2 diabetes

The high sugar content in soft drinks has been linked to an increased risk of developing type 2 diabetes. Regular consumption can lead to insulin resistance, a condition where the body's cells no longer respond effectively to insulin, resulting in elevated blood sugar levels.

Dental issues

Soft drinks, with their high acidity and sugar content, are a major contributor to dental problems. The combination of acid and sugar provides an ideal environment for the growth of bacteria that cause tooth decay. Additionally, the acidity can erode tooth enamel, leading to sensitivity and increased susceptibility to cavities.

Bone health

Phosphoric acid, a common ingredient in many soft drinks, can interfere with calcium absorption in the body. Over time, this can lead to decreased bone mineral density and an increased risk of osteoporosis. This is particularly concerning, especially in adolescents, as it can affect bone development and growth.

Cardiovascular issues

Excessive sugar intake, as seen in regular soft drink consumption, has been associated with an increased risk of heart disease. Consuming too much sugar can lead to elevated blood pressure, inflammation, and unfavourable changes in blood lipid levels, all of which contribute to cardiovascular issues.

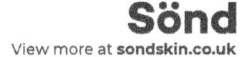

View more at sondskin.co.uk

Insulin resistance and metabolic syndrome

The high fructose corn syrup found in many soft drinks has been linked to insulin resistance and the development of metabolic syndrome. Metabolic syndrome is a cluster of conditions that includes increased blood pressure, high blood sugar, excess abdominal fat, and abnormal cholesterol levels, which collectively elevate the risk of heart disease, stroke, and type 2 diabetes.

Negative impact on mental health

Some studies suggest a potential link between high sugar intake and an increased risk of depression and other mental health issues. The rapid spikes and crashes in blood sugar levels associated with sugary drinks may contribute to mood swings and a decrease in overall mental well-being.

Drink in moderation

It's important to note that moderation is key, and occasional consumption of soft drinks may not lead to significant health issues. However, regularly indulging in these sugary beverages can contribute to a range of health problems, emphasizing the importance of making informed choices about dietary habits. Choosing water, herbal infusions, or other healthier beverage alternatives can be a positive step toward maintaining overall health and well-being.

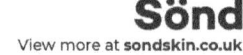

Hidden dangers of energy drinks

In a world that constantly demands high energy and quick solutions, energy drinks have emerged as a popular go-to for individuals seeking an immediate boost.

Marketed as enhancers of alertness, focus, and stamina, these beverages have gained widespread popularity. However, beneath the appealing promises lies a dark side—a myriad of health risks associated with their consumption.

The Caffeine Conundrum

Energy drinks are notorious for their high caffeine content, often far exceeding the levels found in traditional caffeinated beverages like coffee or tea. While caffeine can enhance alertness and concentration in moderate amounts, excessive intake can lead to a range of adverse effects. Insomnia, jitteriness, increased heart rate, and elevated blood pressure are just the tip of the iceberg.

Sugar Overload

Just like their soft drink counterparts, many energy drinks are laden with excessive amounts of sugar or high-fructose corn syrup. Regular consumption can contribute to weight gain, insulin resistance, and an increased risk of type 2 diabetes. The combination of caffeine and sugar may provide a temporary energy spike, but it is often followed by a crash, leaving individuals more fatigued than before.

Cardiovascular Caution

The stimulant properties of energy drinks can have profound effects on the cardiovascular system. Elevated heart rate and blood pressure, coupled with the potential for arrhythmias, pose a significant risk, especially for individuals with pre-existing heart conditions. The surge in adrenaline triggered by energy drinks can lead to a strain on the heart, potentially culminating in serious cardiac events.

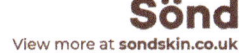

Deceptive Hydration

Despite their widespread use during physical activities, energy drinks are often ineffective at hydrating the body. The diuretic effect of caffeine can contribute to increased urine production, potentially leading to dehydration. This deceptive quality can be particularly dangerous when individuals rely on these beverages during intense workouts or in hot climates.

Mixing Dangers

Energy drinks are frequently combined with alcohol, a practice that can have dire consequences. The stimulating effects of caffeine may mask the depressant effects of alcohol, leading individuals to underestimate their level of intoxication. This dangerous combination can result in risky behaviours, impaired judgment, and an increased likelihood of accidents.

Renal Risks

Prolonged and excessive consumption of energy drinks has been linked to renal issues. The combination of caffeine and other additives may contribute to the formation of kidney stones and potentially impair kidney function over time. These concerns are heightened when individuals consume multiple energy drinks in a short period, leading to a cumulative effect on the kidneys.

How to Navigate the Energy Drink Epidemic

As the consumption of energy drinks continues to surge, it becomes imperative for individuals to be aware of the potential health hazards associated with these seemingly innocuous beverages. From cardiovascular concerns to the hidden perils of excessive caffeine and sugar intake, the risks are substantial.

This chapter serves as a cautionary exploration, urging readers to approach energy drinks with a critical eye and consider healthier alternatives for sustaining energy and vitality. In the quest for a quick energy fix, the toll on health may be far higher than anticipated, and the repercussions could extend far beyond the temporary jolt these drinks provide.

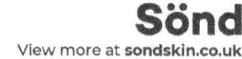

The dynamics of fruit juices

Fruit, a natural source of nutrients and vitamins, offers numerous health benefits. However, its sugar content demands a cautious approach. While fruits are a valuable part of a balanced diet, it's essential to moderate their intake to about 1-2 servings per day, preferably eaten separately from main meals and not consumed after 6 PM, favoring alkaline varieties or consuming acidic ones in smaller quantities.

The benefits of eating whole fruits

Eating whole fruits is preferred over consuming fruit juices. Juicing removes the fiber present in whole fruits, leaving behind concentrated fructose. Fiber plays a crucial role in regulating digestion and promoting a feeling of fullness. Without this fiber, the concentrated sugar content in juices directly impacts the liver and can lead to adverse effects.

Approach smoothies with care

Modern trends have popularized smoothies combining fruits and vegetables. However, it's crucial to maintain a separation between fruit and vegetable smoothies. Opting for vegetable-only smoothies ensures a lower sugar content, supporting a more alkaline environment in the body. Excessive fruit quantities in smoothies contribute to heightened sugar and acidity levels, which may not be beneficial for health.

Commercial bottled juices

Beware of commercially available bottled juices that often contain preservatives, additives, and added sugars, further compromising the nutritional integrity of the juice. The consumption of such bottled juices is discouraged due to their detrimental impact on health.

In essence, the emphasis remains on consuming whole fruits in moderation, prioritizing alkaline options and limiting the intake of acidic fruits. Avoiding the consumption of freshly squeezed fruit juices and steering clear of commercially prepared bottled juices is recommended for maintaining optimal health in an alkaline lifestyle.

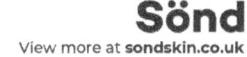

Shopping

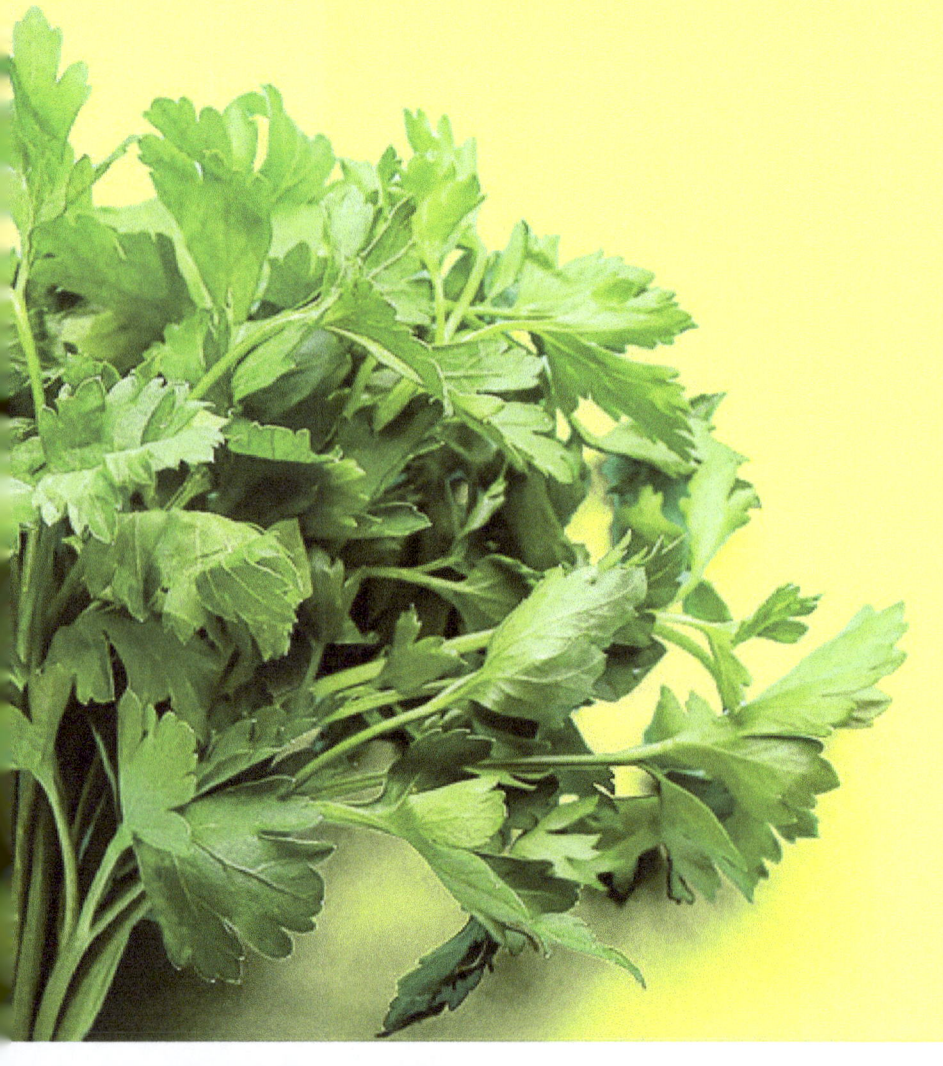

Being mindful of the seasons

Eating seasonal produce provides both more flavour, and higher-quality nutrition. Seasonal produce spends less time getting from farm to table, which allows it to maintain higher nutritional levels and flavour.

When I asked you earlier in this book how green you were, we spoke about the level of greens in your diet. But living an alkaline lifestyle doesn't ignore being green in the environmental sense.

In fact, consuming a diet rich in vegetables, fruits, grains, nuts, and seeds and avoiding or greatly reducing animal-based foods is considered very environmentally friendly as well as being considered healthy.

Our carbon footprint

If we think of our diet in terms of how it impacts greenhouse gas emissions and our carbon footprint, producing plant based foods creates considerably fewer emissions and treads more lightly on Planet Earth than producing meat and dairy products.

Animal feed, animal waste, land use, transportation, and production of animal based products are all very carbon-intensive.

Growing, picking, and preparing plant based foods still has an environmental impact, but it's considerably smaller than that of producing meat and dairy.

So, we can choose to eat more plants in order to make our own environmental impact smaller, but we can go further than that in our quest to look after our own health and that of the environment. Choosing to eat organic plant based produce means that not only are we are consuming food that's free from artificial pesticides and fertilisers, but it also means that the land used to grow them hasn't been contaminated with a cocktail of potentially harmful chemicals.

Seasonal fruit and vegetables

We can also choose to consume seasonal fruit and vegetables, that is, food that's been grown during its natural growing season, such as asparagus in the spring and Brussels sprouts in the autumn and winter.

Seasonal produce is grown, harvested, and transported to our shops without the need for artificial growing conditions (such as polytunnels) or long-term refrigerated storage for future use.

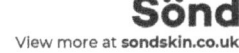

Polytunnels

Polytunnels are made from plastics that perish quickly, need replacing, and also require heating in order to create the warm conditions that spring and summer seasonal produce requires.

They allow produce to be grown all year round, which is great, but they do have a higher associated greenhouse gas emission rate than produce grown outside and in season. Produce grown out of season in artificial growing conditions also needs to be stored in refrigerators or freezers, which themselves have a high environmental cost to run.

Hyper local food

We can't talk about the seasonality of food without also talking about the locality of the food. Locally grown food means food grown in the country it's being eaten in. (Hyper local food is food that's grown within a few miles of where it's being sold and eaten, such as food sold at the farm gate or at local farmers markets.)

Locally grown food has a lower environmental impact (hyper locally grown food even more so) as it doesn't require air freighting or shipping followed by road transport from airports and docks; instead, it'll usually just require road transport.

If a tomato grown seasonally in Spain outside in March reaches our plates here in the UK when it's too early for tomatoes to grow, is it seasonal?

Technically, yes, because of where it was grown, in season. But it isn't local. A tomato grown in the UK in June and then eaten in the UK in June is both seasonal and local.

The nutritional value of food grown seasonally and locally is also considered higher, since nutrients begin to slowly deplete once the food is harvested. However, these nutritional losses are minimal when compared to eating a diet deficient in fresh vegetables.

Therefore, if we're looking for the best and freshest food to consume, then organic, seasonal, locally grown produce is it. But of course this isn't often possible, especially if we're sticking to an alkaline diet full of varied vegetables all year round.

It's important to take a deep breath here and accept that we simply cannot be perfect.

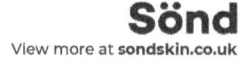

If we choose to drink a green juice for breakfast in the winter and the cucumbers and green peppers have been grown in a Spanish polytunnel and shipped to the UK, we need to make peace with this balance of consuming health-giving foods that still have a lower carbon footprint than animal-based foods, even if the animal has been reared on a farm next door to our home.

Stay mindful

Always be mindful of where your food comes from and how it was produced, and make considered choices as much as time, seasons, availability, and costs allow. But remember, eating seasonally and locally grown produce is just one part of eating sustainably and being mindful of the environment.

Know that we can't be perfect all the time, but we can make choices some of the time that will help. Eating a full or mostly plant based diet overall has a lower carbon footprint than eating animal based foods, so you're already doing well.

If you want to eat more seasonally and locally, it will help to become familiar with the produce that grows seasonally in your area throughout the year.

As a general rule, exotic produce such as papayas and coconuts will always have come from far afield, as they're simply unable to grow in the climate of Northern Europe.

Avoiding pre-prepared, pre-packaged produce such as bagged salads, trimmed vegetables, and chopped fruits will also help to reduce your carbon footprint in terms of processing and single-use plastics.

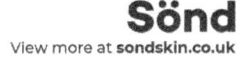

Decoding food labels

In our quest for an alkaline lifestyle and overall well-being, one of the essential skills we must master is deciphering the labels on food products.

It's no secret that many unhealthy and harmful ingredients lurk behind innocent-sounding names, making it crucial for us to be savvy shoppers and informed consumers.

The food industry often employs clever marketing strategies, using ambiguous terms and misleading claims to make their products appear healthier than they truly are.

As health-conscious individuals, we must navigate through these tactics and arm ourselves with knowledge to make wise choices for our bodies and minds.

Scan the ingredient list

The ingredient list is our window into what's really inside the product. Look for transparency and simplicity; the fewer ingredients, the better.

Aim to avoid foods with long lists of unrecognisable additives, preservatives, and artificial colours.

Instead, opt for products with whole, real ingredients that promote alkalinity and support our health.

Watch out for hidden sugars

Sugar is often disguised under various names, such as high-fructose corn syrup, maltose, dextrose, and sucrose.

Keep an eye on these hidden sweeteners, as excessive sugar consumption can lead to inflammation, weight gain, and other health issues.

Choose foods with little or no added sugars and prioritise natural sweeteners like stevia or monk fruit.

Unmask sneaky sodium

Sodium, in excess, can disrupt our body's acid-base balance.

Be wary of sodium-laden ingredients like monosodium glutamate (MSG) and sodium nitrate in processed foods.

Opt for low-sodium or sodium-free alternatives, and season your meals with alkaline herbs and spices.

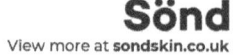

Be cautious with fats

While healthy fats are essential for an alkaline lifestyle, trans fats and hydrogenated oils are harmful.

Keep an eye out for terms like "partially hydrogenated" in the ingredients list, as these indicate the presence of unhealthy fats.

Choose products with good fats, such as avocado, nuts, and olive oil, and avoid those containing harmful fats.

Look for whole grains

Whole grains contribute to alkalinity and provide essential nutrients.

However, not all "whole grain" products are created equal. Ensure the first ingredient is truly whole grain (e.g., whole wheat, quinoa, brown rice) and avoid refined grains like white flour.

Mind the preservatives

Artificial preservatives like BHA, BHT, and sulfites are commonly used to extend shelf life but can disrupt our body's natural balance.

Opt for fresh, whole foods or products with natural preservatives like vitamin E or rosemary extract.

Avoid artificial flavours and colours

Artificial flavours and colours can negatively impact our health and have no place in an alkaline lifestyle.

Choose products with real, natural flavours and colours derived from fruits, vegetables, or herbs.

Empowering ourselves with the knowledge to read food labels will not only aid us in maintaining an alkaline lifestyle but also promote overall health and well-being.

Remember, the best foods are those closest to their natural state, free from harmful additives and processed ingredients. By making informed choices and embracing an alkaline mindset, we can nourish our bodies and live a vibrant, fulfilling life.

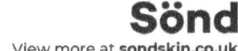

Buying and storing different ingredients

Once fresh vegetables are picked, they quickly begin to lose nutrients. But unless we have a plentiful kitchen garden or allotment that makes us self-sufficient, most of us have to rely on buying our fresh ingredients in shops, supermarkets, and farm shops.

However, we can take steps to protect the nutritional value of the vegetables we buy.

This begins with buying them as fresh as possible and as close as possible to when we intend to eat them. But there are other tips, too, and glass jars are about to become your best friend!

Buying fresh vegetables

The freshest vegetables have the richest colours, flavours and vitality. As much as you can, buy seasonal, locally grown vegetables. Seasonal vegetables are more likely to have been grown in fresh air rather than artificially inside or in polytunnels, and locally grown produce has spent less time travelling from farm to fork, both of which will help to maintain nutritional integrity.

In an ideal world, organic vegetables would be standard, since they contain no traces of pesticides or fertilisers. But organic is often less cost-effective in monetary terms, and sometimes organic options simply aren't available. But where possible, choose organic.

Also, choose vegetables that are loose and not wrapped in plastic. There's still a long way to go in terms of unnecessary single-use plastics and food, but many mainstream supermarkets are now offering a wider range of loose vegetables. Take your own jute or cotton bags to package them up.

Plastics contain BPA and phthalates, which are nasty chemicals that can leach into foods and have been linked to various human health conditions.

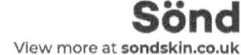

There's been an explosion in zero-waste shops in many towns and cities that offer loose produce as well as dried herbs and spices, beans, legumes, grains, and other store cupboard staples. Visit with your own paper bags and glass jars, fill them, and only pay for what you buy, minus the plastic and waste.

Storing fresh vegetables

However you buy your vegetables, how you store them when you get home is just as vital for preserving nutrients. As soon as you get them home, give all your vegetables a wash in clean, running water.

This helps to remove any dirt and potentially any residues, and it helps them to maintain their vitality and freshness. This, in turn, then helps to nourish and hydrate you better when you eat them.

Once washed, dry them by shaking off the excess water and then dabbing them on paper towels or gently pressing them between two sheets of clean cotton.

Don't overdry them; simply wrap them in absorbent paper towels, put them into a glass jar, and store them in the fridge.

Storing grains and cereals

Dried grains, cereals, beans, and legumes should also be washed at home for a few minutes in a colander with cold, running water. This helps to remove impurities and stickiness when cooked and reduce bitterness.

Before cooking, they should then be soaked overnight in cold water to reduce levels of phytic acid that can interfere with digestibility and nutrient absorption. Place them in a glass bowl and add water to at least 5 cm above the level of the cereals or grains.

Once soaked overnight, rinse them again before cooking according to the packet instructions.

Another helpful tip with cereals is that before adding them to cooking, fry them in a little olive oil for 1 to 2 minutes to help prevent stickiness and glooping and to reduce the nuttiness of their flavour, which can overpower the delicate flavours of vegetables.

Prepared in such a way, they can then be stored in a glass jar for up to five days in a fridge or up to three months in a freezer. All grains, pulses, beans, legumes, dried herbs, spices, and dried fruits can be stored safely in clean glass jars.

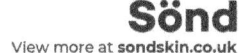

Sprouting seeds and pulses

If you're looking for ways to add even more health and vitality to your alkaline lifestyle, then sprouting is for you. Dried seeds and pulses can all be sprouted, and doing so adds an incredible amount of nutrition in the form of extra vitamins and minerals. Sprouted seeds can then be eaten raw or cooked.

To start the germination process, soak 100 grams of seeds, pulses, or cereals in 250 ml of cold water for 12 hours at room temperature. After 12 hours, drain and rinse well, and transfer to a glass jar covered with a clean cotton cloth secured at the rim with an elastic band. Then, place the jar into a glass bowl at an angle so that the rim of the jar is tilted downward.

Place the bowl away from direct sunlight and continue the process of rinsing, draining, and placing it back into the tilted glass jar every 12 hours. Depending on the seed, you'll start to see the first sprouts form after 1 to 3 days.

Once sprouted, keep them in the glass jar and consume within a few days.

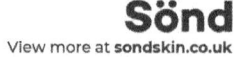

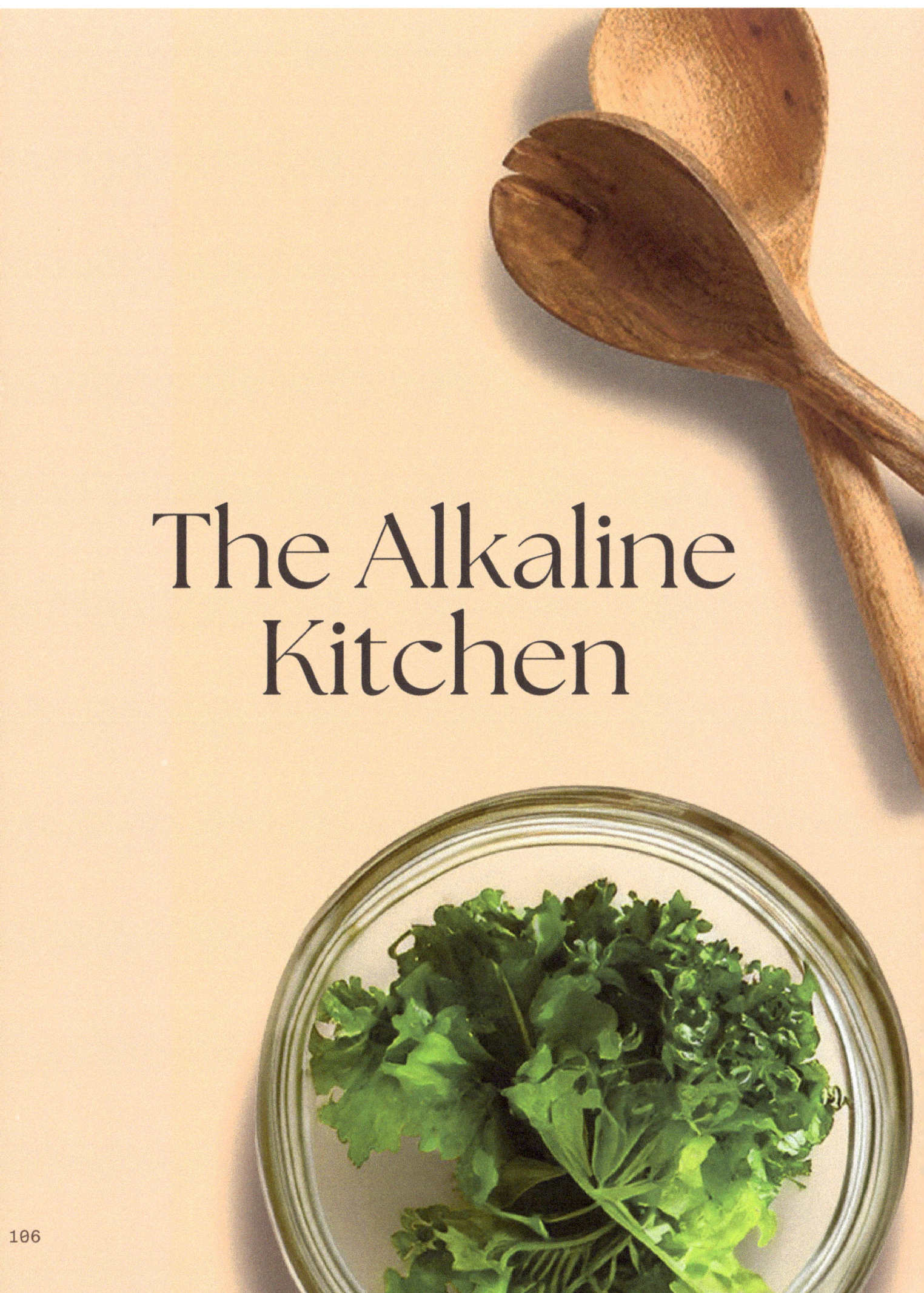

The Alkaline Kitchen

The alkaline kitchen

In the pursuit of an alkaline lifestyle, the kitchen becomes our sanctuary, where we craft nourishing meals to support our well-being.

However, the journey to optimal health goes beyond just the ingredients we use; it extends to the tools we employ in our culinary endeavours.

The right kitchen utensils can enhance the alkaline cooking experience and help us maintain the integrity of nutrient-rich foods.

Let's explore some of the essential quality utensils that align with our alkaline lifestyle:

Stainless steel cookware

When it comes to pots and pans, stainless steel is a top choice for an alkaline kitchen. It's durable, non-reactive, and free from harmful chemicals that can be found in some non-stick coatings.

Stainless steel ensures even heat distribution, preserving the nutritional value of our ingredients while making clean-up a breeze.

Cast iron skillets

Cast iron cookware is a time-tested favourite, not just for its superior heat retention but also for adding trace amounts of iron to our meals.

These skillets are perfect for sautéing vegetables or creating lots of hearty, alkaline-friendly dishes. Be sure to season your cast iron regularly to maintain its non-stick surface.

Glass food storage containers

Properly storing alkaline meals is essential for maintaining their freshness and nutrient content. Glass food storage containers are an excellent choice as they are non-toxic, non-reactive, and free from harmful chemicals found in plastic containers. They also ensure that no unwanted flavours or odours leach into our food.

Bamboo utensils

Embrace eco-friendly utensils with bamboo options. Bamboo is a sustainable material that won't scratch your cookware or leach harmful chemicals into your food. Opt for bamboo spatulas, spoons, and tongs for a natural and alkaline-conscious kitchen.

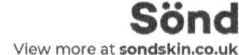

Ceramic knives

When it comes to cutting vegetables and fruits, ceramic knives are a fantastic addition to an alkaline kitchen.

These knives retain their sharpness, are non-reactive, and won't alter the taste of your produce. The precision cutting also helps maintain the integrity of alkaline-rich foods.

High-speed blender

A high-speed blender is an alkaline kitchen's best friend. It effortlessly blends vegetables and leafy greens into smooth, nutrient-packed concoctions. Whether it's a vibrant green smoothie or a creamy soup, a quality blender can be your go-to appliance for creating alkaline delights.

Slow juicer extractor

For those seeking the purest form of nutrient-rich juices, a slow juicer extractor is a definite must-have in the alkaline kitchen.

Unlike high-speed blenders, slow juicers gently extract juice from vegetables without generating heat, preserving essential enzymes and vitamins. The slow extraction process ensures that your juices retain their vibrant colours, flavours, and alkalising properties, making them a delightful addition to your alkaline lifestyle. With a slow juicer extractor, you can enjoy the full benefits of fresh, alkaline-packed juices that nourish your body from the inside out.

Stainless steel strainer

When preparing homemade alkaline nut milks or fresh vegetable juices, a stainless steel strainer is invaluable. It helps achieve a smooth, pulp-free texture, ensuring that all your beverages are easy to digest and bursting with nutrients.

Electric soup maker

It is a convenient kitchen appliance designed to simplify the soup-making process. It combines multiple functions into one device, making it easier and quicker to prepare delicious, homemade soups.

Food steamer

It is a versatile and healthy kitchen appliance that uses steam to cook various types of food. It offers a gentle cooking method that preserves the natural flavours, nutrients, and colours of the ingredients.

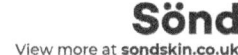

Alkaline water filter

Having access to clean, purified water rich in minerals and electrolytes is crucial for maintaining an alkaline lifestyle. A quality water filter pitcher can remove impurities and toxins, allowing you to enjoy alkaline water that promotes hydration and supports overall well-being.

By equipping our kitchen with quality utensils, we can elevate our alkaline cooking experience and enhance the nutritional value of our meals. These thoughtful choices not only contribute to optimal health but also reflect our commitment to sustainability and holistic well-being.

As we embrace the alkaline kitchen, we nurture a space where health and taste harmoniously blend, fostering a positive impact on our lives and the world around us.

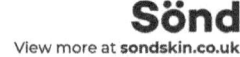

Cooking methods for an alkaline lifestyle

Cooking methods can significantly impact the nutrient content and alkaline properties of the foods we eat.

As we strive to embrace an alkaline lifestyle, it's essential to consider the cooking techniques that preserve the nutritional value of our meals while maintaining an alkaline balance.

In this section, we will explore the differences between various cooking methods and highlight the healthiest options for an alkaline-conscious kitchen.

Microwaving

Microwaving is known for its speed and convenience in preparing meals. However, this cooking method can lead to nutrient loss due to the high heat and short cooking times.

Microwaves can break down vitamins and minerals, reducing the nutritional content of your food.

While microwaving may be suitable for some tasks, such as reheating leftovers, it's best to try to minimise its use for cooking fresh, nutrient-rich foods in an alkaline lifestyle.

Baking or roasting

Baking in the oven is a popular cooking method that can preserve the nutritional integrity of alkaline foods. Unlike microwaving, baking allows for longer, gentler cooking, minimising nutrient loss. Vegetables, grains, and proteins can be oven-baked to perfection, preserving their taste and texture while maintaining their alkaline properties. Using a little healthy fat, like olive oil, during baking can enhance flavour and nutrient absorption.

Grilling and barbecuing

Grilling and barbecuing can infuse foods with smoky and delicious flavours. However, it's essential to be mindful of the potential health risks associated with charring or overcooking. When foods are exposed to high temperatures and direct flames, harmful compounds called heterocyclic amines (HCAs) and polycyclic aromatic hydrocarbons (PAHs) can form, which are linked to cancer risk. To reduce this risk, marinate your alkaline-friendly foods before grilling and avoid prolonged exposure to high heat.

Steaming

Steaming is one of the healthiest cooking methods, especially for an alkaline lifestyle. This gentle process involves cooking food with steam, preserving the natural flavours and nutrients. Steamed vegetables, in particular, retain their vibrant colours and essential vitamins and minerals, making them a perfect addition to an alkaline plate.

Steaming also requires little to no added fat, making it a heart-healthy option.

Stir-frying

Stir-frying is a popular method in many Asian cuisines and offers a balance between quick cooking and nutrient retention. When done right, stir-frying can maintain the alkaline properties of your ingredients while delivering flavourful, colourful meals. Use a healthy oil like coconut or sesame oil and cook over high heat for a short time to maintain the crunch and nutritional value of your alkaline veggies.

Remember, the choices we make in the kitchen contribute significantly to the nourishment and balance we bring to our alkaline lifestyle.

Supplements

The requirement for supplements

The food we choose to eat is directly linked to our physical and emotional health and wellbeing.

If we choose to eat a mostly alkaline diet high in nutritious vegetables and plant-based protein, then we're supporting good health and wellbeing. If we choose to eat a diet high in acid-forming and processed foods, saturated fat, sugar, salt, and protein from animal sources, then we're not treating our body to what it needs.

Nutritional supplements, therefore, have become a 'fix-it' for the latter type of diet. We might take a daily multivitamin supplement each day, telling ourselves that it's undoing all the bad and supplementing our body with what it needs, which is far from the truth. There is no substitute for a healthy, alkaline diet.

However, even if we do eat a mostly plant-based, vegetable-rich, alkaline diet, we still need nutritional help. This is because, unless we're eating a completely organic, biodynamic diet, much of our food, including conventionally grown vegetables, has been interfered with in some way.

Many plants, including vegetables, grains, and pulses, have been grown in the modern way with the use of pesticides, insecticides, and fertilisers (including, in some cases, animal slurry), which not only adds artificial chemicals but also interferes with our nutrient absorption.

Add to that a stressful, busy life, exposure to environmental pollutants and toxins, the occasional takeaway, or even skipping a meal altogether, and we can see the need for high-quality nutritional supplements. Most of the time, when we think of nutritional supplements, we think of vitamins, but minerals are just as important.

A good-quality supplement that contains a variety of vitamins and minerals and no unnecessary fillers and excipients, such as talc, is therefore a good idea.

However, they should be seen as supplementary to an otherwise healthy, balanced, and nutritious diet, not as a replacement for good-quality food.

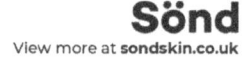

Bio-availability is important

As well as taking a supplement free from chemical fillers, bioavailability is important—that is, how well the nutrients within a supplement can be absorbed and assimilated by the body. Some nutrients have low bioavailability, such as vitamin C, which is a water soluble vitamin.

As you may know, oil and water don't mix well, and water soluble vitamin C will struggle to absorb into the cell membranes as they're made from fat soluble fatty acids.

So this is where liposomal supplements are helpful.

Liposomal supplements

A liposome is a nanometre-sized, ball shaped structure with a water based, hollow centre and an outer shell made from phospholipids (lipid is the chemical name for fat).

Discovered in the 1960s, liposomal encapsulation technology was a breakthrough in the problem of getting certain oral medicines and supplements through the gut and into the bloodstream.

The hollow centre can be filled with medicine or a nutritional supplement such as vitamin C, and the result is the most bioavailable type of supplement.

Liposomal supplements have an outer membrane that's chemically similar to that of our own cellular membranes, meaning that liposomal supplements can move across cell membranes more efficiently to ultimately deliver their nutrients to the cells where they're needed.

This clever outer membrane also protects the nutrients inside the liposomal supplement as they pass through the acidic conditions of the stomach and the digestive enzymes produced by the liver so that they can arrive at the cells via the bloodstream, intact.

A daily liposomal supplement is therefore another pillar of your alkaline-based approach to natural wellbeing.

Speak with a professional nutritionist

Taking supplements can be beneficial for filling nutritional gaps and supporting your overall health. However, it's crucial to make informed choices. Before selecting any supplements, it's wise to consult your family doctor. They can assess your health condition and review your blood test results to determine which specific nutrients you may be lacking and in what quantities. This personalised approach ensures that you're taking supplements that align with your individual needs and contribute positively to your well-being.

Your doctor's guidance is essential for a safe and effective supplementation plan.

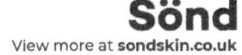

The healing potential of sea-derived supplements

Supplements derived from sea algae, such as seaweed or algae-based supplements, can be beneficial in supporting an alkaline lifestyle due to their nutrient-rich profile and unique healing properties.

Here are some ways in which sea algae supplements can help:

Rich in alkalising minerals

Sea algae are abundant in essential minerals such as calcium, magnesium, potassium, and iron, which are all alkaline-forming in the body. These minerals help balance the body's pH levels and contribute to maintaining an alkaline state.

Antioxidant support

Sea algae are a source of various antioxidants, including vitamins C and E, beta-carotene, and phytonutrients. Antioxidants help neutralise free radicals, reducing oxidative stress and inflammation, which can contribute to acidity in the body.

Algae-based omega-3 fatty acids

Some sea algae supplements provide essential omega-3 fatty acids, particularly DHA and EPA, which are typically found in fish oil.

Algae-based omega-3s offer a plant-based alternative to fish-derived omega-3s, and they have anti-inflammatory properties that can support an alkaline lifestyle.

Detoxification support

Sea algae contain natural compounds that support the body's detoxification processes. By aiding in the elimination of toxins and heavy metals, sea algae can help reduce the acidic burden on the body.

Digestive health

Certain types of sea algae, such as spirulina and chlorella, contain dietary fiber that supports a healthy digestive system. A well-functioning digestive system ensures efficient nutrient absorption and waste elimination, which contribute to overall alkalinity.

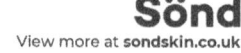

View more at sondskin.co.uk

Supporting the immune system

Sea algae contain various compounds, including polysaccharides and peptides, that can strengthen the immune system. A robust immune system helps the body fight off infections and maintain optimal health, contributing to an alkaline state.

Enhancing energy and vitality

The nutrient density of sea algae can provide a natural boost of energy and vitality, making it easier to stay active and engage in physical activities, both of which are essential components of an alkaline lifestyle.

Minimising acidic food choices

Incorporating sea algae supplements can be a helpful strategy to balance the diet, especially for those who may occasionally consume acidic foods. By providing alkaline-rich nutrients, sea algae supplements can offset the acidity of other dietary choices.

It's important to note that while sea algae supplements can be a valuable addition to an alkaline lifestyle, they should not be considered a substitute for a well-balanced alkaline diet based on fresh fruits, vegetables, whole grains, and plant-based proteins. Supplements should complement a healthy diet and lifestyle rather than replace essential nutrients obtained from whole foods.

Taking supplements can be beneficial for filling nutritional gaps and supporting your overall health. However, it's crucial to make informed choices. Before selecting any supplements, it's wise to consult your family doctor. They can assess your health condition and review your blood test results to determine which specific nutrients you may be lacking and in what quantities. This personalised approach ensures that you're taking supplements that align with your individual needs and contribute positively to your well-being. Your doctor's guidance is essential for a safe and effective supplementation plan.

The health benefits of brown algae

Brown or bitter algae are a crucial and valuable component of an alkaline diet, primarily due to their exceptional nutrient profile. These marine plants, commonly found in seawater environments, offer a plethora of health benefits that align perfectly with the principles of an alkaline lifestyle.

High mineral content

One of the key attributes of brown algae is its high mineral content. They are an abundant source of essential minerals such as calcium, magnesium, potassium, and iron.

These minerals play vital roles in various physiological processes, including bone health, nerve function, muscle contraction, and the maintenance of proper electrolyte balance.

Moreover, brown algae are rich in vitamins, particularly vitamin K and several B-vitamins, which are essential for energy production, blood clotting, and the health of the nervous system. Additionally, these seaweeds contain significant amounts of valuable vitamin C, a potent antioxidant that supports the immune system and combats oxidative stress.

Brown algae are renowned for their unique polysaccharides and fibers, which have prebiotic properties that nourish beneficial gut bacteria. A healthy gut microbiome is crucial for overall well-being, as it is linked to improved digestion, enhanced nutrient absorption, and even a strengthened immune system.

Furthermore, brown algae boasts a remarkable content of bioactive compounds, including polyphenols and phlorotannins, which exhibit powerful antioxidant and anti-inflammatory properties. These compounds help protect our cells from damage caused by free radicals, reduce inflammation, and promote overall cellular health.

Incorporating brown or bitter algae into an alkaline diet can be highly beneficial, contributing to a balanced and nutrient-rich eating regimen. Whether enjoyed in culinary dishes, as a supplement, or in various culinary creations, these seaweeds offer a fantastic way to boost your alkaline lifestyle and support your body's overall health and vitality. So, don't hesitate to explore the world of brown algae and embrace their goodness as a delightful addition to your alkaline journey.

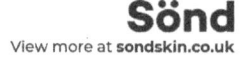

Due to their ability to absorb harmful substances from the marine environment, bitter algae serve as excellent natural detoxifiers.

When consumed, they can perform the same function within our bodies, aiding in the elimination of accumulated toxins and improving the health of the digestive system.

High in fiber and antioxidants

Bitter algae are a valuable source of dietary fiber, promoting regular bowel movements and supporting digestive health. Additionally, they contain potent antioxidants like fucoxanthin, which combat oxidative stress and help protect cells from damage caused by free radicals.

Immune system support

Packed with vital nutrients, including vitamins, minerals, and essential amino acids, bitter algae can support and strengthen the immune system. A robust immune system is crucial for preventing diseases and infections and maintaining overall body balance.

Weight management aid

Bitter algae are characterised by their high fiber content and low caloric value, making them an excellent choice for those looking to maintain or achieve a healthy weight. The fiber slows the absorption of sugars and fats, promoting satiety and helping to control appetite.

Bitter algae are a treasure of nature that offer numerous health benefits and seamlessly complement an alkaline lifestyle. Incorporating them into your diet will allow you to harness their beneficial properties and enjoy radiant health and overall well-being.

Indeed, the strong taste of bitter algae can be a deterrent for some individuals when considering their consumption. However, this should not discourage anyone from benefiting from their valuable nutrients. For those who find it challenging to include bitter algae in their diet, taking algae-based supplements is an excellent alternative.

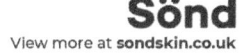

Brown algae supplements

Supplements provide a convenient and efficient way to enjoy the varied and plentiful health-enhancing properties of bitter algae without dealing with the taste. These supplements often come in various forms, such as capsules, tablets, or powdered extracts, making it easy to incorporate them into daily routines.

However, it's essential to exercise caution when consuming bitter algae supplements, particularly if you have specific medical conditions. Individuals with hyperthyroidism, a condition characterised by an overactive thyroid gland, should avoid consuming excessive amounts of seaweed, including bitter algae. Seaweeds naturally contain iodine, which can interfere with thyroid function in individuals with this condition.

Additionally, some antidepressant medications may interact with the iodine content of bitter algae. If you are taking antidepressants or have any medical concerns, it is best to consult with a healthcare professional before incorporating bitter algae supplements into your routine.

By being mindful of these considerations and taking appropriate precautions, bitter algae can become an invaluable addition to an alkaline lifestyle, supporting overall health and well-being.

Whether through dietary intake or supplementation, embracing the benefits of bitter algae can be a transformative step toward achieving an alkaline lifestyle and optimizing your quality of life.

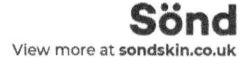

Alkaline Skincare

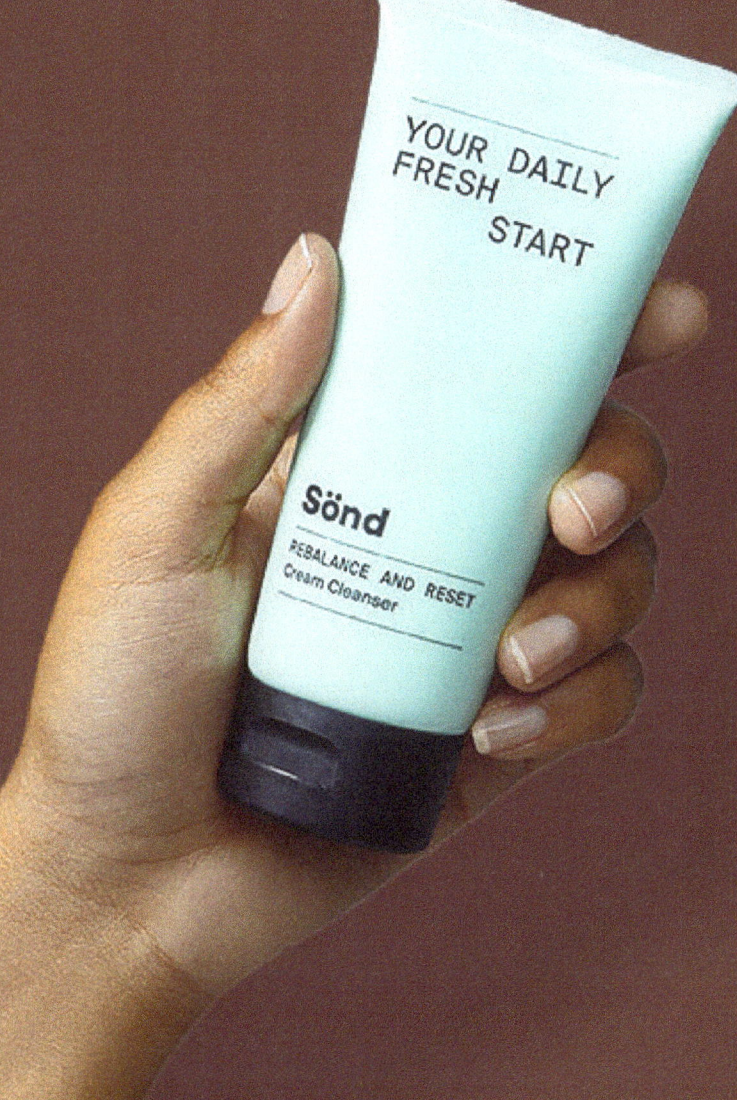

The power of alkaline skincare

Until now, most of what I've discussed and advised in this book has been related to the many benefits of an alkaline-based approach to natural wellbeing for our bodies **on the inside**.

But **our outside** deserves just as much attention, and after all, our skin is our largest organ.

It forms the first part of the immune system, acting as a physical barrier to microscopic and physical invaders alike (along with the few well-guarded weak points discussed previously, such as the mucosal immune system).

Deep within the lower layers of the skin, the skin's regeneration and healing processes are hard at work, providing a continual turnover of new skin cells that move up through the layers, arriving at the surface to replace the dead skin cells that are then naturally shed from the skin.

Skincare products therefore need to be able to penetrate deep into the skin to nourish, hydrate, and support these processes. But not all of them do.

At this level, the skin is naturally alkaline, around pH 7.3, which allows skin cells to thrive and maintain their optimal health. The problem is that most skincare products have an acidic pH of around 5.5.

Applying acidic skincare products to our skin is therefore unhelpful for allowing the skin to thrive, glow, and look healthy. They may support the upper layers of skin that have a slightly acidic pH, but they don't support the deeper layers, where nourishment and hydration are most important for healthy cell renewal.

That's why I encourage the use of deeply penetrating, alkalising skincare made using natural ingredients and alkalising silica salts, with no unnecessary chemicals such as parabens, phthalates, and detergents to get in the way.

Alkalising skincare products help to maintain the natural pH of the deeper layers of skin, which in turn places the cells under less stress. It also provides them with the trace elements they need for maintenance and the elimination of toxins.

Using alkaline skincare products helps to support the natural barrier function of the skin, along with encouraging hydration and the production of the proteins collagen and elastin that keep the skin plump, supple, and youthful.

Sönd

Sönd is a fantastic skincare brand that specialises in alkalising products, including a cream cleanser, hydrating serum, day and night moisturiser, oils and a refreshing toner.

Their alkaline skincare products have been developed to suit all skin types, especially those with skin that's prone to oiliness, dryness, acne, or inflammation. It also deeply hydrates, helps to keep the skin supple and youthful by minimising the signs of ageing and is ideal for the face as well as the neck and décolletage.

A simple, twice-daily skincare routine using Sönd products to support, nourish, and hydrate the skin will help to keep your skin happy and healthy.

Find out more about Sönd here:

www.sondskin.com

Dry brushing

Dry brushing is the highlight of an alkaline routine. It's something to look forward to each morning, especially when using the Dry Brush. With fine bronze bristles made from copper and tin, using this brush provides a satisfying tingling sensation to the skin that helps to invigorate both the body and mind upon waking. The special makeup of the bristles means that oxygen ions are stimulated within the skin and are then readily available for metabolism.

Adding two to three minutes of dry brushing using a body brush with added copper bristles to your morning routine will help to stimulate blood flow and introduce special oxygen ions into the body. Oxygen ions are charged with energy, which is transferred to the body, helping to revitalise it after a night's sleep.

Dry body brushing also helps to oxygenate the skin and connective tissues, improve muscle tone, reduce cellulite, and assist the lymphatic system in draining away excess fluids and toxins. It also brightens and tightens the skin and removes dead skin cells.

How to use a dry brush

Each morning, before your cold shower, brush your body using small circular clockwise motions with gentle pressure. Always work towards your heart, starting at the bottom of your right leg and moving upwards towards your groin, then repeat on your left leg.

Do the same on your right arm, moving towards your armpit, and follow with your left arm. Then gently brush your stomach upwards towards your chest and then up towards your neck. If you can, bush your back using the same circular motions, starting at the base and moving upwards. A partner may come in handy here if you can't reach!

Avoid brushing over sensitive areas, inflamed skin, broken capillaries, or varicose veins. Brushing towards your groin and armpits helps to support the work of the lymphatic system, encouraging the natural movement of lymph fluid towards the lymph nodes.

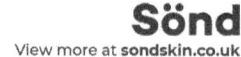

Eliminate toxins with an alkaline bath

An alkaline bath can be a beneficial addition to a detoxification or self-care routine, as it may help eliminate toxins and support overall health.

The idea behind an alkaline bath is to raise the pH level of the water, making it more alkaline than the body's natural pH, which is slightly acidic.

Here are some potential benefits and the importance of an alkaline bath for toxin elimination:

Detoxification

The skin is the body's largest organ and plays a significant role in detoxification. When you soak in an alkaline bath, it may help draw out toxins from the skin through a process called reverse osmosis. Toxins and impurities can then be released from the skin into the alkaline water.

Balancing pH levels

An alkaline bath can help balance the body's pH levels by neutralizing acidity on the skin's surface. Some proponents of alkaline baths believe that maintaining a slightly alkaline pH on the skin can support overall health and reduce inflammation.

Relaxation and stress relief

Like any warm bath, an alkaline bath can promote relaxation and stress relief. Reduced stress levels are beneficial for the body's natural detoxification processes and overall well-being.

Skin health

An alkaline bath may help improve the condition of the skin by promoting a more balanced pH and reducing inflammation. It can be especially beneficial for individuals with skin conditions like eczema or psoriasis.

Muscle recovery

Soaking in an alkaline bath with added alkaline, such as epsom salts or magnesium, can aid in muscle recovery after physical activity. Magnesium is known for its ability to relax muscles and reduce muscle soreness.

Improved circulation

Warm water can promote blood circulation, which helps deliver oxygen and nutrients to the body's cells. Improved circulation can enhance the body's natural detoxification processes.

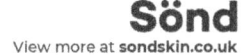

Enhanced hydration

Some proponents suggest that alkaline water may be better absorbed by the skin, which can contribute to enhanced hydration and improved skin health.

While an alkaline bath can be a relaxing and potentially beneficial practice, it's essential to remember that the body's natural detoxification organs, such as the liver and kidneys, are the primary means of eliminating toxins. An alkaline bath should be viewed as a complementary practice to support overall well-being, but it should not replace a healthy lifestyle, a balanced diet, and regular exercise.

How to enjoy an alkaline bath

To create an alkaline bath, you can add alkaline substances like baking soda, Epsom salts, or alkaline bath salts to warm bathwater. Follow the recommended usage instructions for the specific product you choose.

As with any new wellness practice, consult with a healthcare professional if you have any underlying health conditions or concerns.

Daily lymph drainage exercises

n a similar way that our circulatory system allows the circulation of blood through a network of blood vessels, our lymphatic system runs throughout the major tissues of the body, allowing the passage of lymph.

Lymph is a fluid that surrounds the cells and tissues and carries lymphocytes, a type of white blood cell that forms part of the immune system. It also drains away excess fluid, delivers nutrients to the cells, and transports cellular waste, bacteria, and toxins to the bloodstream, where they'll be delivered to the liver and kidneys to be filtered away from the body in the urine.

Lymph fluid flows around the body via a network of lymph vessels that are connected via several lymph nodes, most notably in the neck, armpits, abdomen, and groin, and lymph tissues including the tonsils, spleen, and thymus gland.

Since it carries lymphocytes, the lymphatic system forms an important part of the immune system, assisting the blood in delivering important white blood cells to where they're needed to fight and defend against infection.

The lymphatic system is also responsible for fluid balance within the body, taking excess fluid from the spaces between the cells called interstitial spaces and placing it back into the bloodstream once it's been filtered by the lymph nodes.

Our bodies are remarkably good at allowing the lymphatic system to get on with balancing fluids, filtering, delivering nutrients, supporting the immune system, and removing waste. However, sometimes the system can become blocked, particularly if we develop an infection, causing the lymph nodes to swell if they encounter excess foreign materials and toxins.

A blocked or sluggish lymphatic system can result in lethargy, weight gain, backache, and constipation.

Lymph drainage exercise

There is a simple everyday exercise that helps to support the work of the lymphatic system, helping to release any blockages and allow the normal passage of fluids, nutrients, and waste throughout the body.

To perform a lymphatic drainage exercise, simply lie on your back with your hands held together on the floor above your head. Slowly raise your legs until they're at right angles to your body, and keep your ankles together.

Remain in this position for at least ten minutes and complete it three times a day. By performing this exercise, you're allowing gravity to help drain the lymph fluid from the lower half of your body to aid it in its journey to the major organs in your torso.

Make this part of your daily practice, and you'll be supporting your lymphatic system, the drainage of toxins and waste from your body, and helping to strengthen your immune system.

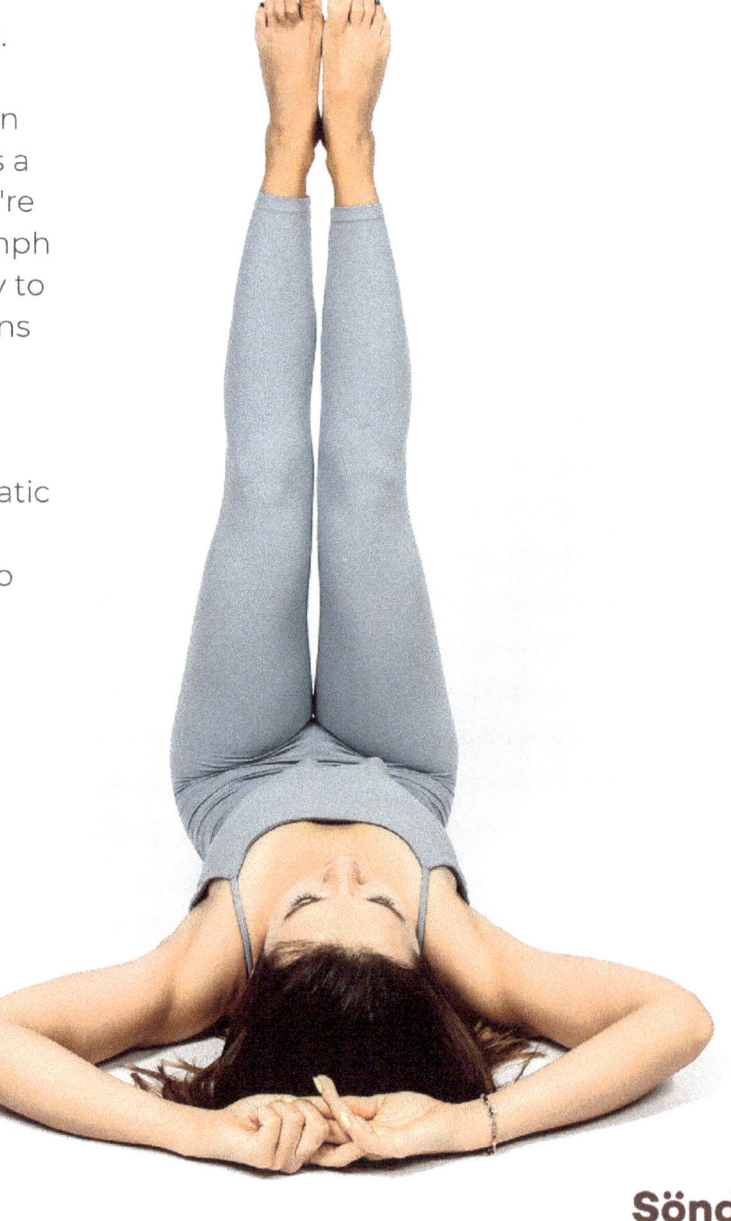

Algae-based facial treatments

Facial treatments with algae can be a valuable addition to an alkaline lifestyle, offering various benefits for skin health and overall well-being.

Algae, particularly seaweed, is rich in nutrients, minerals, and antioxidants that can support skin hydration, nourishment, and rejuvenation.

Here are some ways algae-based facial treatments can complement an alkaline lifestyle:

Skin hydration

Algae extracts are well known for their ability to lock in moisture and improve skin hydration.

Properly hydrated skin appears plumper, smoother, and more radiant, which aligns with the goals of an alkaline lifestyle focused on overall health and well-being.

Nutrient-rich

Algae is packed with vitamins, including vitamins A, C, E, and B, as well as essential minerals like magnesium, calcium, and zinc. These nutrients are essential for healthy skin and can help support its natural repair processes.

Antioxidant protection

Algae contains a wide range of antioxidants, such as beta-carotene, phycocyanin, and flavonoids, which help protect the skin from oxidative stress and free radicals. Antioxidants are crucial for maintaining youthful skin and reducing signs of ageing.

Detoxification

Algae extracts have detoxifying properties that can help draw out impurities and toxins from the skin. Detoxified skin is better able to absorb nutrients and maintain its natural balance.

Soothing and calming

Algae-based facial treatments can have a calming effect on the skin, reducing inflammation and redness. This can be particularly beneficial for those with sensitive or irritated skin.

Improved skin elasticity

Algae extracts can promote collagen synthesis, which supports skin elasticity and firmness. This can contribute to a more youthful and lifted appearance.

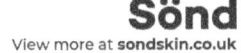

Brighten and even skin tone

Some algae species contain compounds that can help to brighten the skin and even out skin tone, reducing the appearance of dark spots and hyperpigmentation.

Reduced puffiness

Algae treatments can help reduce puffiness and swelling, especially around the eyes.

This can contribute to a refreshed and rejuvenated appearance.

Relaxation and stress relief

Like any other facial treatment, an algae-based facial often includes massage techniques that promote relaxation and reduce stress. Managing stress is vital for maintaining an alkaline state and overall well-being.

It's important to note that while these algae-based facial treatments can offer numerous benefits, achieving an alkaline lifestyle requires a holistic approach that includes a balanced diet, regular exercise, stress management, and adequate sleep.

When considering algae facial treatments, it's essential to consult with a licensed esthetician or skincare professional who can recommend the most suitable treatment based on your skin type and concerns.

Additionally, opt for reputable spas or skin care clinics that use only the best high-quality algae products to ensure safety and efficacy.

Overall, incorporating algae-based facial treatments into an alkaline lifestyle can provide a nourishing and rejuvenating experience for the skin, contributing to a healthy, radiant complexion.

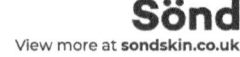

Algae-based body treatments

Algae-based body treatments can play a supportive role in an alkaline lifestyle by providing various benefits to the body and skin.

Algae, particularly seaweed, is naturally alkaline and contains an abundance of minerals, vitamins, and antioxidants that can complement the alkaline diet and promote overall well-being.

Here are some ways algae body treatments can help enhance an alkaline lifestyle:

Detoxification

Algae, being rich in chlorophyll and other detoxifying compounds, can help the body eliminate toxins. Algae body wraps, baths, or scrubs can assist in drawing out impurities from the skin and promoting lymphatic drainage, which supports the body's natural detoxification processes.

Skin nourishment

Algae is packed with nutrients that can nourish the skin, including vitamins A, C, E, and minerals like magnesium, calcium, and zinc. Regular algae body treatments can provide essential nutrients to the skin, supporting its health and radiance.

Hydration

Algae is known for its ability to retain moisture, making it beneficial for maintaining skin hydration. Properly hydrated skin can appear more plump and youthful, contributing to a more vibrant appearance.

Cellulite reduction

Some algae body treatments are targeted at reducing cellulite. The minerals and compounds in algae can help improve circulation, reduce inflammation, and break down fat cells, which may contribute to a reduction in the appearance of cellulite.

Skin tightening and firming

Algae-based body treatments can help improve skin elasticity and firmness, contributing to a more toned appearance.

Relaxation and stress relief

Many algae body treatments are accompanied by massages, which can promote relaxation and reduce stress. Lowering stress levels is important for maintaining an alkaline state, as chronic stress can lead to increased acidity in the body.

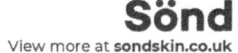

Improved blood circulation

Algae treatments that involve massage or body wraps can enhance blood circulation, which supports the delivery of nutrients and oxygen to the skin and body tissues.

pH balancing

While algae itself is alkaline, the specific effect on the body's pH from topical application during body treatments may be limited. However, the overall benefits of these treatments can contribute to better skin health and overall well-being, which aligns with the goals of an alkaline lifestyle.

It's important to note here that while algae-based body treatments can be beneficial, they are not a substitute for a well-balanced alkaline diet and a healthy lifestyle.

Adopting an alkaline lifestyle involves consuming nutrient-rich, alkaline foods, staying hydrated, exercising regularly, managing stress, and getting enough good quality sleep.

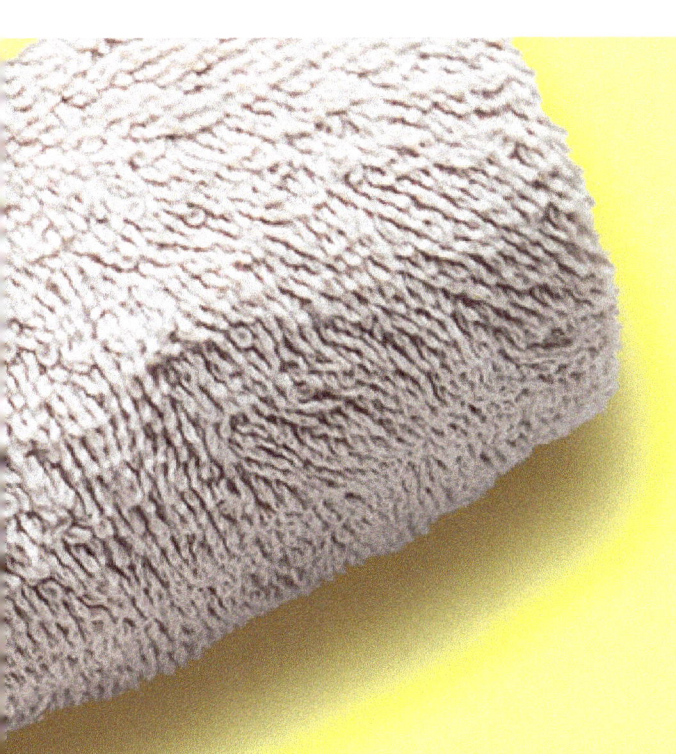

Alkaline Lifestyle

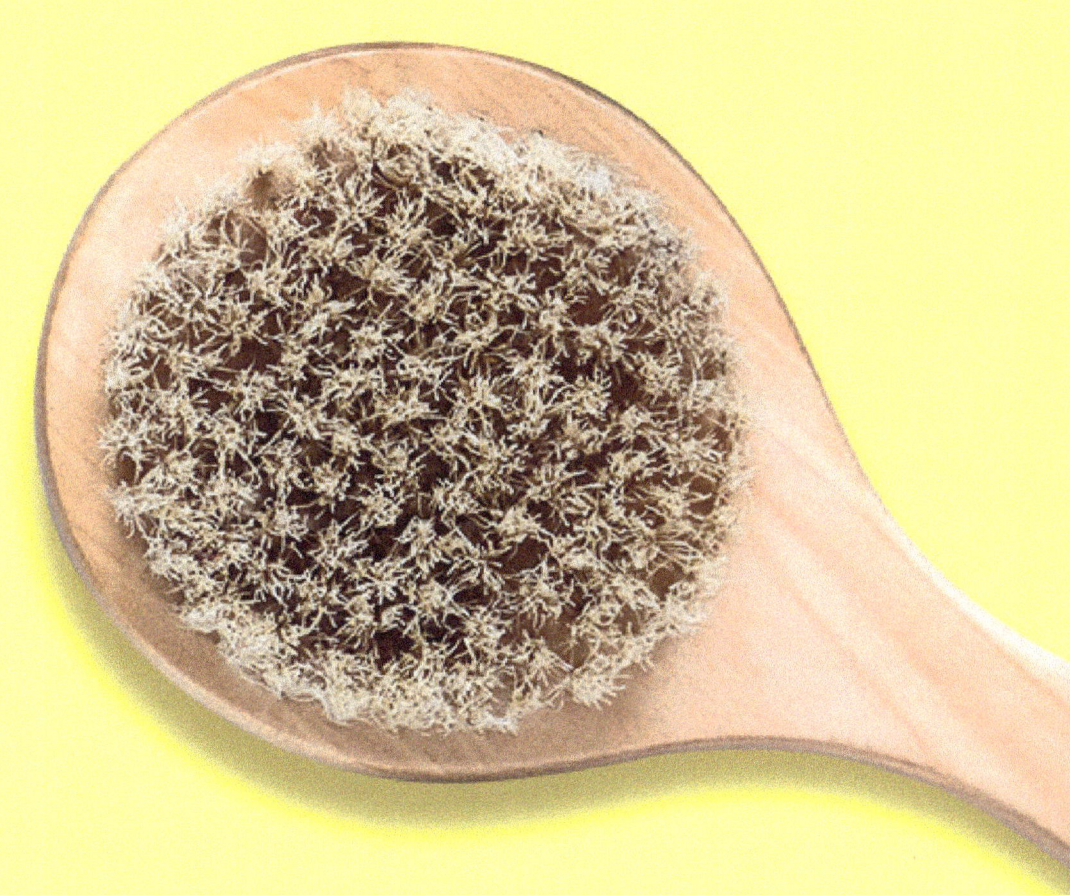

An important daily routine

As you might expect, an alkaline-based approach to natural wellbeing is more than just consuming an alkaline diet; there are lifestyle adaptations too. Practising them regularly and making them part of your everyday routine will soon become second nature.

An alkaline-based daily routine looks like this:

- Daily dry body brushing using a brush with copper bristles
- A daily morning shower protocol
- The use of alkaline skincare products twice a day
- Lymph drainage exercises three times a day
- Practising correct breathing techniques
- Achieving good-quality sleep
- Taking liposomal supplements every day

As with any aspect of adapting to an alkaline lifestyle, the key is to take things slowly.

Don't try to change everything at once, and always be gentle with yourself if you miss one or two aspects of your alkaline daily routine.

As with the 80:20 rule of alkaline eating, the point is to add these to your daily routine most of the time. Trying to change your lifestyle, exercise, sleep patterns, and skincare all at once might feel overwhelming, which can mean that we become more inclined to give up completely.

So I suggest taking one or two and perfecting them for a week or so, then introducing more. You may find that you already have some perfected. For example, you may already achieve good-quality sleep, or you may already use alkaline skincare products. Either way, getting to the point where all of these aspects become a daily habit will help you achieve your goal of health, wellness, and balance.

Concentrate first on what you've added to enrich your life, then think about what you need to remove in order to support an alkaline lifestyle.

Celebrate every achievement, confident in the knowledge that any change you make is more than you've done until this point.

In the chapters that follow, I'll go over the other important aspects of your daily alkaline routine, why they're beneficial, and tips on achieving them.

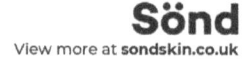

The benefits of a cold shower

What if I told you that a cold shower each morning is about to become part of your alkaline lifestyle? I expect you'd shudder. But showering in cold water has unique benefits for our overall health and wellness, especially the health of our immune system.

The importance of having a strong immune system

The immune system is a complex system of cells, molecules, tissues, and organs that work tirelessly together to help protect us against disease and infection.

It's our first line of defence against intruders, including cold and flu viruses, vomiting bugs, bacterial infections, and even a splinter in our finger.

Having a compromised immune system, caused in part by a poor diet, high levels of stress, smoking, drinking excessive amounts of alcohol, and living a sedentary lifestyle, can mean that we become more susceptible to illnesses and infections. We become unwell more often, seemingly catching every bug that's doing the rounds. We become lethargic, unproductive, unmotivated to exercise, and make unhealthy life choices, making us more unwell. It's a vicious cycle.

Eating nutritious foods, spending time in fresh air, doing regular gentle exercise, taking steps to reduce stress, staying well hydrated, and getting enough good quality sleep all help to support a strong, healthy immune system. This will result in more energy, fewer infections, and a quicker recovery when we do succumb to illness. But there's one more thing we can add to that list: a daily cold shower.

The benefits of cold showers

Cold showering isn't a new concept, but it's risen in popularity in recent years thanks to Dutchman Wim Hof. Motivational speaker, adventurer, and extreme athlete, it's safe to say Wim is a fan of the cold.

With world records for prolonged full-body contact with ice and ice swimming and being a regular barefoot half marathon runner over ice and snow, he's well respected in the field of cold therapy.

Wim is able to endure extremely cold temperatures as he's trained his breathing so much that it controls his heart rate and blood circulation, meaning he's able to survive such extreme conditions.

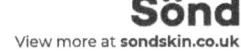

Through his controlled breathing techniques and beliefs, he's been able to scale some of the highest and coldest mountains on earth wearing just a pair of shorts, withstand two hours immersed in ice, and run a marathon in the hot, arid conditions of the Namib Desert without stopping for any water.

The Wim Hof Method

He's developed the Wim Hof Method, a method of breathing that allows advocates to gain a greater awareness of their breath and to learn how to manipulate their breathing to their advantage. It also utilises the benefits of cold therapy, and the two are tied together with a personal commitment to master the breathing techniques and withstand the cold.

The three "powerful pillars" of the Wim Hof Method—cold therapy, breathing, and commitment—are the basis of the method and, once mastered, can lead to exceptional benefits.

I'm going to talk in more detail about breathing in another chapter in this section, but cold therapy is something I want to introduce you to now, and it forms a major part of an alkaline lifestyle.

Regular exposure to the cold brings multiple benefits, including an increase in the 'good fat' of the body, otherwise known as brown adipose tissue, thermally active tissue that produces more heat and increases the metabolic rate, leading to increased fat and calorie burning potential.

Cold therapy can also benefit the immune system by reducing inflammation within the body, helping to keep our hormones balanced, improving our sleep quality, and boosting our mood by releasing feel good endorphins.

White blood cells called lymphocytes form an important part of the immune response. For example, if we cut ourselves, lymphocytes will flood the area to help defend an open wound against bacteria and viruses that could cause it to become infected. Lymphocytes are also present in large numbers around the mucous membranes, such as our nostrils and mouth, which serve as openings to the inside of the body (the respiratory and gastrointestinal tracts, respectively), where invading pathogens could gain entry. (This is known as the mucosal immune system.)

The lymphocytes are better able to travel in the bloodstream to where they're needed if our blood flow, or circulation, is healthy and unimpeded.

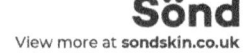

Cold showers improve our circulation and therefore improve the ability of our immune system to work to defend us against illness and disease.

But cold water therapy isn't simply a case of stepping into a cold shower and trying to withstand the shock for as long as possible. It takes time to learn the process and to slowly build stamina.

How to take a cold shower

A cold shower should only be used when your body is warm, so upon waking, it is ideal. Set your shower to a warm to hot temperature (around 35 to 38 °C; this is probably your usual, go-to shower setting). Stand under the water until you feel that your body is well warmed. You can soap your body during this time too.

Then, turn the water temperature down to lukewarm (around 20 to 23 °C, which should feel noticeably cooler). You can gradually work your way towards 15 to 18 °C, which will feel distinctly cold. Make sure your shower head is on a jet setting rather than a waterfall-type setting, and then, holding the shower attachment, shower your body in the following order:

- The outer side of your right leg, starting at your foot, rising to your hip, and then the inner side of the same leg, from your thigh to your foot
- Repeat the process on your left leg
- The outer side of your right arm from the back of your hand to your shoulder and back, then from your armpit down the inside of your arm to your palm
- Repeat the process on your left arm
- The top of your back down to your buttocks
- Your chest down to your stomach
- Your neck up to your face

The entire process should be repeated twice and should last around ten minutes. Perform this daily, and your immune system will soon be reaping the benefits.

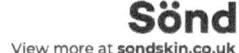

The importance of good quality sleep

How do you feel after a night of interrupted sleep?

Tired, irritable, unable to concentrate, and willing for the day to end so that you can return to bed?

That's the story for most of us after a night of tossing and turning, broken sleep, and hours of wakefulness when it feels like our brain just won't switch off.

If we achieve better sleep the following night, then we're normally re-set and able to get on with normal life. But if we consistently get poor quality sleep or not enough sleep, then our health can be significantly impacted. In fact, a chronic lack of sleep is responsible for a wide variety of physical and mental health symptoms that can negatively impact our quality of life.

Physiological functions

When we sleep, our physiological functions, such as breathing and digestion, slow down. Our temperature and blood pressure drop, and our cells undergo a process of regeneration. Our brain also stores away all the memories and thoughts from the day. So it's clear that sleep is important, both in terms of quality and quantity.

Ideally, adults aged 26 to 64 should aim for between seven and nine hours each night, with no fewer than six or more than ten. Young adults should aim for the same, but with no fewer than six or more than 11 hours, and the elderly between seven and eight hours, achieving no less than five and no more than nine hours of sleep.

It is advisable to go to bed before midnight, regardless of your age, to ensure that you receive adequate rest and recovery.

A chronic lack of sleep can lead to poor cognitive skills such as learning, concentration, and memory, mood swings, and impaired decision making, leading to risky behaviour.

It can increase our risk of experiencing accidents, cause us to become more at risk of chronic diseases such as heart disease and type 2 diabetes, and even cause us to gain weight.

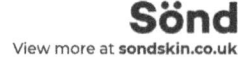

The many risks associated with a chronic lack of sleep

Sleep is beneficial for our emotional wellbeing; we only need to think about our moods when we're tired to know that. If we struggle to sleep on a regular basis, our concentration, performance, and productivity will all also struggle, as will our ability to reason and solve problems.

We'll be less inclined to make healthy choices too, such as choosing to exercise or eat well. In fact, a lack of sleep can lead to obesity, as tiredness can lead us to consume extra calories in the form of comfort foods and refined carbohydrates.

Poor sleep quality can also interfere with the hunger hormones ghrelin and leptin, which will make us feel hungry more often and take longer for us to feel full.

Exercise

If we do find the energy to exercise, we might find that our tiredness makes our regular exercise more difficult, meaning that we don't fulfil our potential by performing fewer reps or running at a slower pace.

This can cause frustration and lead us to simply give up exercising altogether. We might also be more at risk of injury if we have poor form.

Long term impacts

In terms of our physical health, spending less time asleep can increase our risk of developing type 2 diabetes, and not just because we might be more prone to gaining weight or becoming obese.

A chronic lack of sleep can interfere with our glucose metabolism, leading to insulin resistance, which in turn can lead to prediabetes and type 2 diabetes. Insulin resistance and type 2 diabetes are associated with metabolic disease, which can increase our risk of developing heart disease and strokes too.

Chronic inflammation is also associated with a higher risk of disease and can be caused by a poor or acid-forming diet, smoking, stress, and an unhealthy lifestyle. But a lack of good quality sleep can also cause inflammation, which in turn can add to the vicious cycle of chronic disease and an impaired immune system.

Finally, a chronic lack of sleep can lead to a reduction in our ability to keep our emotions balanced, to interact on a social level with family members, friends, peers, and strangers, and to a low mood and depression.

It's therefore crucial, for all aspects of our health and wellbeing, that we do all we can to get enough good quality sleep on a regular basis.

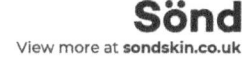

Tips to improve your sleep hygiene

Achieving enough good quality sleep can sometimes be difficult, especially if we're under a lot of stress or we have a baby (or puppy!) that's keeping us awake. But there are things we can do to improve our so-called "sleep hygiene"—the habits we have that can support or hinder our sleep.

- Make sure your bedroom is cool, dark, quiet, well-ventilated, and free from clutter.
- Playing a sleep meditation or white noise as you get into bed can help you drift off.
- A weighted blanket can help promote deep sleep by providing a feeling of support; opt for a breathable one made from bamboo or organic cotton rather than polyester, especially if you're a hot sleeper.
- Try to stick to the same wake-sleep times, even at weekends, to support your circadian rhythms or internal body clock.
- Take steps to reduce stress, such as mindfulness and yoga practice.
- Avoid using smartphones and tablets in the hour before bed, as they emit blue light that tricks the brain into thinking it's daytime.
- Avoid vigorous exercise or a large meal too late into the evening, as both are stimulating.
- If you consume caffeine, avoid drinking caffeinated drinks past lunchtime.
- Avoid alcohol in the hours before bedtime; it may send you to sleep, but you'll miss out on important REM sleep.
- Smoking is the ultimate health no-no, even for sleep. If you smoke, seek help from your doctor or pharmacist to begin quitting.
- Make sleep an important pillar of your well-being, and don't neglect it in favour of another chapter or episode of your current box set or scrolling aimlessly through social media.

Achieving good quality sleep and enough of it is just as important to our overall wellbeing as a healthy diet, regular exercise, and staying hydrated.

Being busy, coping with stress, and our social lives and life in general can get in the way of a healthy sleep pattern, but I hope that following my sleep hygiene tips will help if you struggle with your sleep.

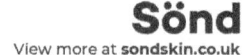

Mastering a good breathing technique

Breathing is something that we all do subconsciously without giving it too much thought. Yet it's critical to life.

Although we'd be weak and uncomfortable, we could survive a few days without water and a few weeks without food. But most of us can only survive a minute or two without breathing. We're constantly breathing, and it's automatically controlled by the autonomic nervous system, so we don't have to think about it. But we should be thinking about our breath in order to optimise our health.

So right now, take a moment to pause and focus on your breathing. Are you breathing slowly or at a faster pace? Are you taking long, slow, deep breaths or quick, shallow breaths?

During practices that encourage us to focus on our breath, we're encouraged to breathe deeply and slowly, but that isn't the full story. If you regularly practice mindfulness meditation or yoga, you'll know that focusing on the breath is important for emotional wellbeing and focus. But do you know how to breathe for proper wellbeing?

The correct technique

The correct mindful breathing technique can help us achieve incredible benefits for our mind and body. Such breathing techniques are one of the best ways to lower our stress and anxiety levels and allow our body to become more alkaline. When we breathe deeply, our brain receives messages to pause, calm down, and relax. The brain then sends this message to our body, and we unwind. Yet most of us are unaware that something as simple as correct breathing can make such a difference, and we instead spend our lives breathing incorrectly.

For example, when we're crossing the street at a green light and a car suddenly appears at speed, what do we do? We quickly inhale and move fast in order to escape. This is a sympathetic nervous system response, as opposed to our regular autonomic nervous system-controlled breathing, and is a perfectly acceptable breathing reaction, given the circumstances. In other words, it's our fight-or-flight response.

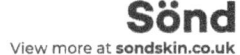

But what if I told you that most people breathe in this same way all of the time? As if we're about to be hit by a car all day long, every single day? It sounds exhausting, doesn't it? But for many, it's a reality without even knowing it.

So I'll invite you once more to reflect on your breath right now. Are you breathing slowly or at a faster pace? Are you taking long, slow, deep breaths or quick, shallow breaths?

The benefits of breathing correctly

Breathing is the biological process of taking in air, absorbing the oxygen from it so that it can be transported around the entire body, and then breathing out carbon dioxide. (Incidentally, trees and plants do the opposite; they use carbon dioxide for photosynthesis and release oxygen, so while we breathe in their oxygen, they're using our carbon dioxide—a beautiful example of symbiosis in nature.)

The more oxygen we introduce into our bodies as we inhale, the more energy is available to our cells for chemical and biological processes. If we optimise our breathing, it can significantly impact our health.

Learning how to master good breathing techniques can offer incredible benefits to both our mind and body and improve our quality of life by:

- Reducing depression
- Reducing stress levels
- Lowering our heart rate
- Lowering our blood pressure
- Improving diabetic symptoms
- Improving our management of chronic pain
- Better regulating our body's reaction to stress and fatigue

But it isn't just about how much oxygen we inhale; carbon dioxide levels are just as important.

Carbon dioxide

When we think about breathing, we tend to place emphasis on the importance of oxygen. Oxygen is certainly important; it plays a role in everything from cellular function and repair to digestion, brain function, and muscular contraction. But carbon dioxide, often considered a 'waste product' of digestion, is equally as important. It's used for the dilation (widening) of the arteries and airways, the elimination of waste products, and, amazingly, an increase in the absorption of oxygen.

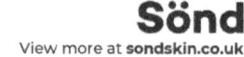

Yogic breathing teaches us that the balance of these two gases is ideal and that the ultimate goal of correct breathing techniques is to manipulate the levels of carbon dioxide in the bloodstream and lungs rather than the level of oxygen.

If we breathe slowly, we increase the level of carbon dioxide in the blood, meaning that our oxygen saturation (level of oxygen in the blood) is lower. But this doesn't mean that there's less oxygen in the body. In fact, when we have an increase in carbon dioxide achieved through slow, meaningful breathing, we increase the level of oxygen absorption in our cells.

We can demonstrate this: if we breathe quickly, then we don't increase our cellular oxygen as expected, and we feel dizzy from a lack of oxygen as we're not maintaining the balance of carbon dioxide to oxygen.

So we need to breathe more slowly in order to conserve carbon dioxide and increase our cellular oxygen level.

Breathe through your nose

Yoga breathing also teaches us that, crucially, breathing should occur through the nose, both inhalation and exhalation, rather than exhaling through the mouth. When we breathe through our nose, we add nitric oxide to our breath.

Nitric oxide is a powerful bronchodilator and vasodilator, which means that it widens the breathing tubes and blood vessels, respectively. It's essential for the health of the blood vessels and the heart and for good circulation.

Try to practice correct breathing at a certain point each day—slow, mindful, deep breaths. Set a timer or use a mindfulness app with guided meditation. Practice for a little longer each day until your 'normal' breathing is slow and purposeful.

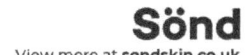

Breathing techniques that benefit health

Mastering the art of breathing can lead to remarkable improvements in our well-being. Various breathing techniques offer unique advantages, impacting our overall well-being.

Different nostril breathing

The different nostril breathing technique, which utilizes alternating nostrils, serves as one powerful method.

The human body experiences a nasal cycle where one nostril is dominant over the other. Breathing primarily through the left nostril is associated with a calming effect due to the parasympathetic activity that promotes relaxation. Conversely, the right nostril is linked to an energizing effect and increased sympathetic activity, resulting in a more alert state. The nasal cycle typically alternates every few hours throughout the day, allowing each nostril to take turns in dominance for breathing.

This nasal phenomenon can be utilized in breathing techniques. By closing one nostril, an individual can direct their breath through the other nostril. For instance, breathing through the left nostril may induce relaxation, while breathing through the right nostril might prepare the body for action. These techniques can be used to help regulate energy levels and manage stress in various situations.

Additionally, distinct breathing practices adopted at various times of the day provide unique benefits. Understanding and leveraging these techniques can significantly impact our daily lives, allowing us to harness the power of our breath for better health and vitality.

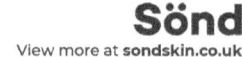

Morning "Coffee" breathing - Breath of Fire

This technique, primarily practiced in the morning, is particularly notable for its capacity to increase pH levels in the body, fostering a more alkaline environment.

As you begin, ensure you are in a comfortable position while lying down. Close your eyes and allow your chin to remain parallel to the floor. Relax your face and shoulders. This exercise serves to wake up and energize the body. To practice, start by exhaling sharply, engaging the muscles of your lower abdomen, and creating a sensation similar to a sneeze. Following the forceful exhale, relax and allow the inhalation to occur naturally. Focus on these strong, sharp exhales and let the inhalation happen in a relaxed, effortless manner.

Performing the described sequence for three rounds of 20 breaths each.

"Water" Breathing - 4:4 Balance Breathing

This technique is adaptable for use at any time during the day. It is versatile and aids in relaxation and stress reduction.

This breathing exercise is also known as "4:4 Balance Breathing". It promotes a balanced and steady breathing pattern, facilitating relaxation and harmony.

Start comfortably seated with your eyes closed, chin parallel to the floor, and keep your face and shoulders relaxed. Ensure that you breathe exclusively through your nose. Maintain a consistent rhythm: a 4-count inhale followed by a 4-count exhale.

Performing the described sequence for one round of 10 breaths each.

With your eyes still closed, allow your breath to return to its natural rhythm, free from any counting – simply let it flow naturally.

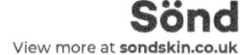

Whiskey Breathing - 4:8 Relaxation Technique

This breathing exercise is designed for bedtime and is done after you've laid down in bed.

Begin by lying down on your back. Position your right hand on your chest and your left hand on your abdomen. Keep the right hand stationary while the left-hand rises and falls with each breath during the exercise. Close your eyes to start. Extend the duration of the exhale, doubling the time. Inhale for a count of 4 and exhale for a count of 8. This breathing pattern enhances the relaxation response, and the goal is to manage the exhale slowly to avoid expelling air too quickly.

Rest your hands at your sides in a relaxed manner. Keep your eyes closed. Breathe naturally. Sweet dreams !!!

The importance of exercise

Exercise plays a crucial role in an alkaline lifestyle, contributing to overall health and well-being. When combined with an alkaline diet, regular physical activity can have a profound impact on maintaining the body's acid-base balance and promoting optimal health. Here are some of the key reasons why exercise is an important part of an alkaline lifestyle:

Aids detoxification

Exercise promotes sweating, which helps eliminate toxins from the body. This process supports the body's natural detoxification pathways, allowing for the removal of acidic waste products and metabolic by-products.

Enhances circulation

Physical activity improves blood circulation, ensuring that oxygen and nutrients are efficiently delivered to cells throughout the body. Proper circulation helps support cellular metabolism and waste removal, contributing to a balanced pH level.

Reduces inflammation

Regular exercise has anti-inflammatory effects on the body. Chronic inflammation is associated with an acidic internal environment, and by reducing inflammation, exercise helps support a more alkaline state.

Supports bone health

Weight-bearing exercises, such as walking, running, or resistance training, promote bone density and strength. This is essential for maintaining the body's mineral balance and preventing the release of calcium from bones, which can contribute to acidity.

Improves insulin sensitivity

Physical activity enhances insulin sensitivity, allowing the body to regulate blood sugar levels more effectively. Stable blood sugar levels are associated with a more balanced pH environment.

Boosts immune function

Regular exercise has been shown to enhance immune function, which helps the body defend against infections and maintain overall health. A strong immune system can support the body's ability to neutralise acidic waste.

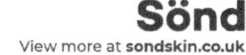

Promotes stress reduction

Exercise is a natural stress reliever, reducing cortisol levels and promoting a sense of well-being. High stress levels can contribute to acidity in the body, so managing stress through exercise is beneficial for maintaining alkalinity.

Supports weight management

Regular physical activity helps manage body weight and body fat levels. Excess body fat can lead to increased inflammation and acidity, so maintaining a healthy weight is important for an alkaline lifestyle.

Improves digestion

Exercise stimulates the gastrointestinal tract, promoting healthy digestion and regular bowel movements. Efficient digestion helps prevent the accumulation of acidic waste in the body.

Supports mental health

Exercise has numerous mental health benefits, including reducing anxiety and depression. A positive mindset and mental well-being are essential for overall health and maintaining an alkaline lifestyle.

When incorporating exercise into an alkaline lifestyle, it's essential to choose activities that you enjoy and can sustain over time.

Aim for a combination of cardiovascular exercises, strength training, and flexibility exercises to achieve a well-rounded fitness routine.

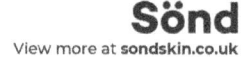

Biofilia for vitality and wellbeing

In our fast-paced, technology-driven world, it's easy to feel disconnected from nature. However, deep within each of us lies an innate longing to be surrounded by the natural world. This longing is known as "biophilia," an instinctual affinity for living organisms and nature. As we explore the intersection of biofilia and the alkaline lifestyle, we discover a profound connection that can significantly enhance our quality of life.

Numerous studies have shown that immersing ourselves in natural environments can have a profoundly positive impact on our physical and mental well-being.

Time spent in nature has been linked to reduced stress levels, improved mood, better immune function, and enhanced cognitive abilities. By incorporating biofilia into our daily lives, we can support the body's natural healing processes and further amplify the benefits of an alkaline lifestyle.

One of the key elements of an alkaline lifestyle is maintaining an optimal pH balance in the body.

Nature, in its abundance, offers us a treasure trove of alkaline-rich foods such as fresh vegetables, fruits, and greens.

By developing a close relationship with nature through biofilia, we become more attuned to the nourishing gifts it provides. By harvesting and consuming these alkaline foods, we nourish our bodies from within, promoting a balanced pH and supporting overall health.

Incorporating biofilia into our daily routine allows us to slow down, practice mindfulness, and embrace the beauty of our surroundings. Whether it's taking a leisurely walk in the park, gardening, or simply sitting under a tree, these mindful moments in nature enable us to disconnect from the stresses of modern life. The practice of biofilia encourages us to be present in the moment, cultivating a sense of inner peace and tranquility that complements the serenity of an alkaline lifestyle.

Biofilia not only involves connecting with nature but also designing our living spaces to reflect the natural world. By integrating natural elements like plants, natural light, and earthy colors, we create an environment that promotes well-being and fosters an alkaline-friendly atmosphere. A biofilic home or workspace can have a positive impact on our mood, productivity, and overall health, making it an ideal complement to our alkaline journey.

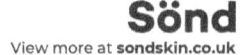

In our bustling urban environments, it's easy to feel detached from nature. However, incorporating biofilia into our lives can help bridge this gap, allowing us to maintain a balance between the demands of modern life and our connection to the natural world.

By spending time outdoors, choosing alkaline-rich foods, and designing biofilic spaces, we create a harmonious ecosystem that supports our alkaline lifestyle and enriches our quality of life.

In a world that often pulls us away from nature, embracing biofilia can be a transformative journey toward an enriched alkaline lifestyle. By nurturing our connection with the natural world, we open ourselves to a wealth of health benefits and a sense of profound well-being.

So, let us embark on this journey together, cultivating our bond with nature and reaping the rewards of a balanced and vibrant alkaline lifestyle.

Biofilic harmony with nature

The term "biophilia" refers to the innate human connection and affinity for nature and living organisms.

Embracing biophilia and incorporating it into your alkaline lifestyle can have several positive effects on your overall well-being and adherence to the alkaline principles.

Here are some ways in which biophilia can enhance your alkaline lifestyle:

Encouraging plant-based nutrition

Biophilia fosters a deeper appreciation for plants and their role in our ecosystem. This appreciation may lead to a stronger inclination towards plant-based nutrition, which aligns perfectly with an alkaline lifestyle. Emphasising fresh fruits, vegetables, leafy greens, and herbs in your diet helps alkalise the body and provides essential nutrients.

Mindful eating

Practising biophilia involves being present and mindful in nature. This mindfulness can extend to your eating habits. By being more aware of the source and quality of your food, you may make better choices that align with the alkaline diet's principles, such as opting for organic and locally sourced produce.

Stress reduction

Spending time in nature and fostering a biophilic connection has been shown to reduce stress and promote relaxation. Stress can contribute to acidity in the body, so incorporating biophilic practices like walking in nature, gardening, or simply spending time outdoors can help manage stress and support your alkaline lifestyle.

Physical activity

Biophilia often involves engaging in outdoor activities that promote movement and exercise. Regular physical activity is essential for maintaining a healthy body and supporting an alkaline lifestyle.

Whether it's hiking, biking, or simply enjoying a walk in the park, these activities contribute to your overall alkaline well-being.

Better sleep

Exposure to natural light and fresh air, both common in biophilic practices, can positively impact your circadian rhythm and improve sleep quality. Sufficient and restful sleep is crucial for overall health and helps your body maintain an alkaline balance.

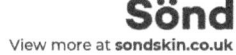

View more at **sondskin.co.uk**

Connection with seasonal foods

Embracing biophilia can deepen your connection with the changing seasons and the foods they offer. Seasonal foods tend to be fresher, more nutrient-dense, and aligned with the body's needs throughout the year, supporting your alkaline lifestyle goals.

Environmental awareness

Biophilia fosters a sense of environmental consciousness and responsibility. This awareness can extend to making eco-friendly choices in your diet, such as reducing food waste and opting for sustainable packaging, which complements the alkaline lifestyle's focus on natural, wholesome foods.

A holistic approach to health

Biophilia promotes a holistic view of health, recognising the interconnectedness of humans with nature. This perspective aligns with the holistic principles of the alkaline lifestyle, which emphasises overall well-being and the importance of nurturing both the body and the environment.

Incorporating biophilia into your alkaline lifestyle can create a powerful synergy that not only enhances the health benefits of the alkaline diet but also nurtures a deeper connection with nature and the world around you.

By embracing biophilic practices and adopting an alkaline lifestyle, you can experience improved physical health, mental well-being, and a greater sense of harmony with the natural world.

The dark side of blue light

In this digital age, we are constantly surrounded by electronic devices emitting blue light.

From our smartphones and laptops to LED screens, blue light has become an integral part of our daily lives. However, its prevalence raises concerns about its potential negative effects on our health and well-being.

In this chapter, we explore the dark side of blue light and its impact on our physical and mental health.

What is blue light?

Blue light is a short-wavelength, high-energy light that is part of the visible light spectrum. It is naturally present in sunlight and plays a crucial role in regulating our sleep-wake cycles and overall circadian rhythm.

However, with the advent of modern technology, artificial sources of blue light have become prevalent, exposing us to higher levels of blue light than ever before.

One of the most significant concerns associated with blue light exposure is its effect on our sleep patterns.

Blue light suppresses the production of melatonin, the hormone responsible for inducing sleepiness.

Prolonged exposure to blue light, especially before bedtime, can disrupt our circadian rhythm and lead to difficulty falling asleep and poor sleep quality.

Staring at screens for prolonged periods can cause eye strain, discomfort, and dryness. This condition, known as digital eye fatigue or computer vision syndrome, is exacerbated by blue light emitted by digital devices.

Studies suggest that prolonged exposure to blue light may contribute to macular degeneration, a leading cause of vision loss in older adults. Blue light exposure may cause damage to the light-sensitive cells in the retina over time.

Some research indicates that excessive exposure to blue light may contribute to mood disorders such as depression and anxiety. The disruption of our natural sleep-wake cycle can lead to changes in mood and cognitive function.

Emerging evidence suggests that blue light exposure at night may be linked to an increased risk of certain chronic health conditions, including obesity, diabetes, and cardiovascular diseases.

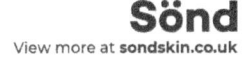

Mitigating the negative effects of blue light

- Many electronic devices now come with built-in blue light filters or "night mode" settings that reduce the amount of blue light emitted. Enabling these features during the evening hours can help protect our sleep.
- Limiting screen time, especially before bedtime, can help reduce blue light exposure and promote better sleep.
- Blue light-blocking glasses are designed to filter out or reduce the amount of blue light reaching our eyes, helping to alleviate eye strain and fatigue.
- Establishing a nighttime routine that involves dimming lights, reducing screen time, and engaging in relaxing activities can signal our bodies to prepare for sleep.

To reduce the effect of blue light and its impact on our bodies, you can incorporate the following plants near your computer or electronic devices:

- **Aloe vera** is not only known for its soothing properties for the skin but also for its ability to absorb indoor pollutants, including formaldehyde and benzene. Having an Aloe Vera plant near your computer can help improve the air quality and create a more refreshing environment.
- **Snake plants (Sansevieria)** are excellent air purifiers that can help remove toxins from the air, including formaldehyde, benzene, and xylene. They are easy to care for and can thrive even in low-light conditions, making them ideal for office spaces.
- **Spider plants (Chlorophytum comosum)** are known for their air-purifying abilities, effectively removing pollutants like formaldehyde and xylene. They are low-maintenance and can thrive in indirect light, making them suitable for indoor settings.
- **Peace lilies (Spathiphyllum)** are beautiful, low-light plants that can help filter out indoor air pollutants such as ammonia, formaldehyde, and benzene. They also add a touch of elegance to any workspace.
- **Boston ferns (Nephrolepis exaltata)** are great at humidifying indoor spaces and can help reduce airborne pollutants. They prefer indirect light and thrive in humid conditions, making them suitable for offices with air conditioning.
- **Bamboo palms (Chamaedorea seifrizii)** are effective at removing formaldehyde, benzene, and trichloroethylene from the air. They require bright, indirect light and can liven up your workspace.

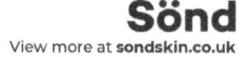

- **Rubber plants (Ficus elastica)** are known for their ability to purify the air and remove pollutants like formaldehyde. They prefer bright, indirect light and can add a touch of greenery to your desk or office space.

- **Dracaena plants (Dracaena spp.)** come in various varieties and are excellent at filtering out indoor air pollutants. They thrive in moderate to bright light conditions and can be a cosy addition to your workspace.

Remember to place these plants within a reasonable distance from your computer to create a more balanced and soothing environment.

While plants can help mitigate the effects of blue light, it's still essential to practice screen time management and incorporate other blue light reduction strategies to protect your overall health.

An important note

I hope you enjoyed this book as much as I did creating it, and I hope that you're now ready to embrace your alkaline lifestyle.

It's important for me to point out that I don't offer individualised medical advice or prescribe any treatments. This also refers to any form of conversation between myself and any of my readers or website visitors.

None of my advice or recipes in this book are a prescription or meant to diagnose or treat any medical condition. Nor do they make any claims to make specific health improvements. Health is a complicated puzzle, of which food and diet are only one piece. If you have any known allergies or intolerances to any of the ingredients used in this book, or you suspect you might have, then avoid those ingredients.

If you have a concern over your health, speak to your GP or another medical practitioner who can discuss your individual case and medical history with you and advise you on the best course of action.

The information contained within this document is for informational and educational purposes only. It's not an attempt by the writers or the publisher to diagnose or prescribe, nor should it be construed to be such. The sources used have been deemed reliable, but no guarantees, expressed or implied, can be made regarding the accuracy of the same. Therefore, readers are also encouraged to verify, for themselves and to their own satisfaction, the accuracy of all reports, recommendations, conclusions, comments, opinions, or anything else published herein before making any kind of decision based upon what they have read. If you have a medical condition, please consult your medical practitioner.

This book is the work of Dr. Anna Brilli in partnership with Sönd Wellbing Ltd. You don't have the right to reprint, sell, auction, or distribute this work. You're not allowed to give away, sell, share, or circulate this work or its content in any form. Books and electronic books are protected under international copyright and intellectual property law. Copyright infringement and theft of intellectual property are serious crimes.

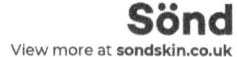

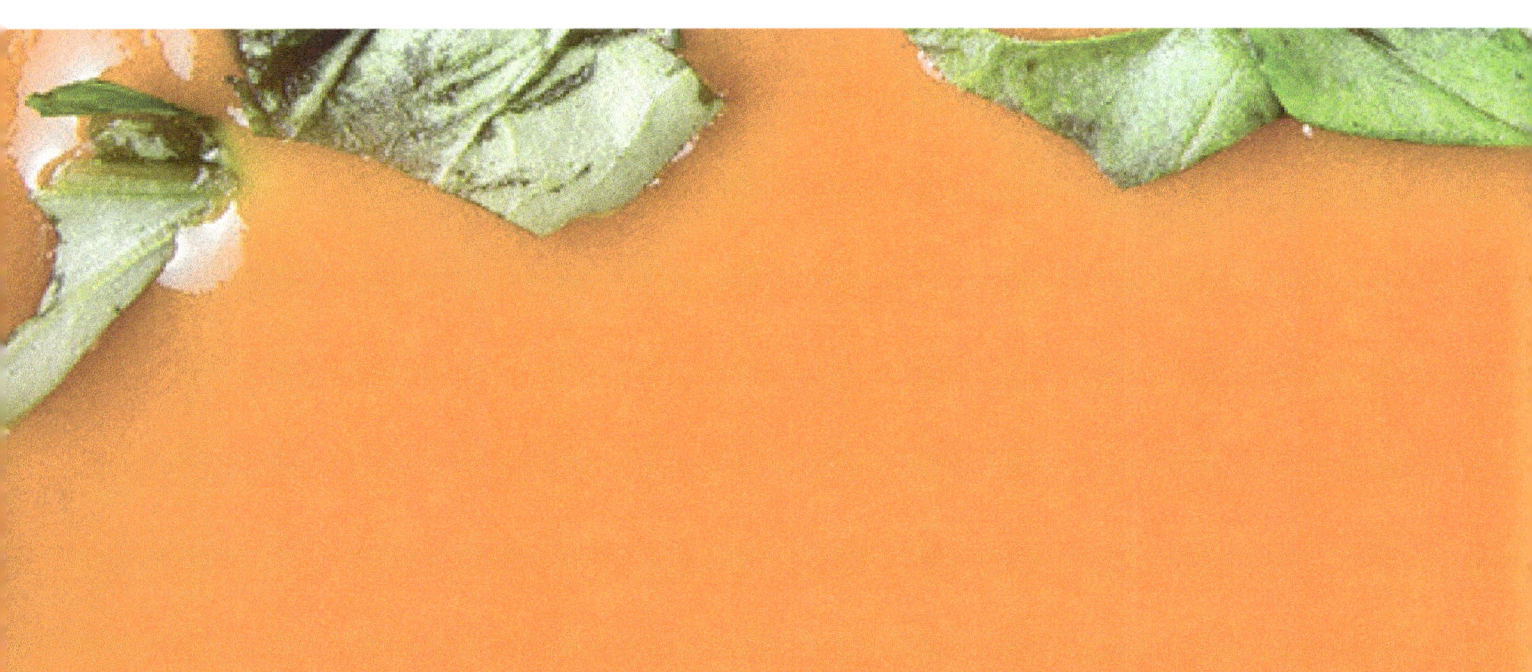

Detox Week Plan, Shopping List & Recipes

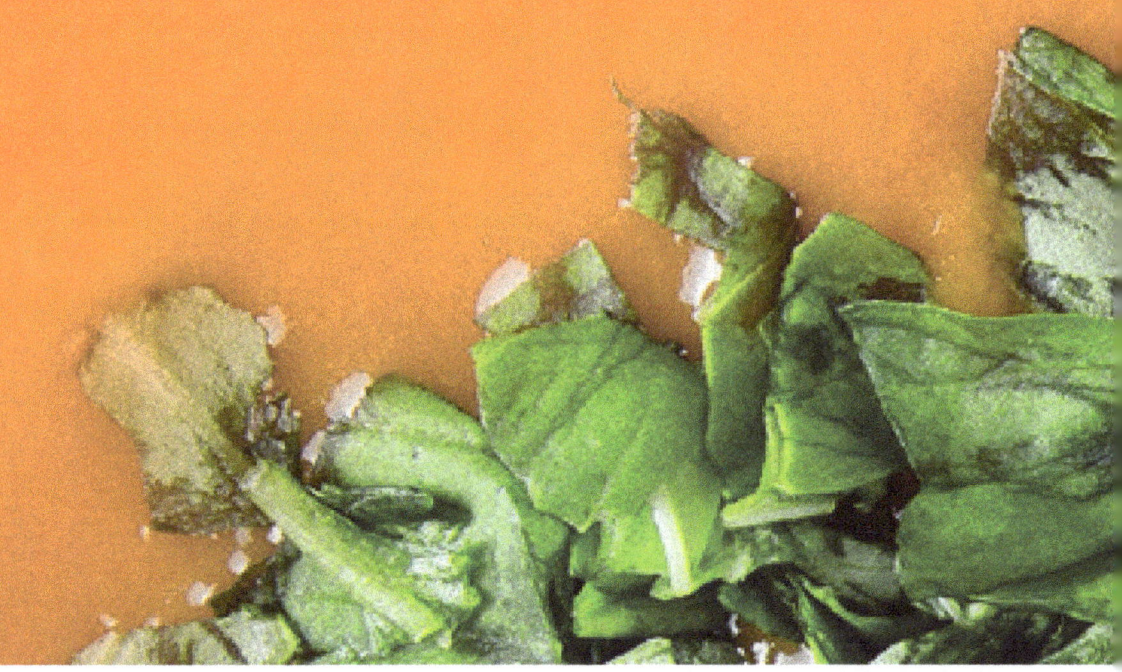

7-Day Detox Meal Plan

	Upon waking	Before Breakfast	Breakfast	Snack	Lunch	Snack	Dinner
Sunday	Lemon tea	Red juice	Gazpacho	Red juice	Carrot, coriander and sesame seeds	Red juice	Gazpacho Green artichoke and bean soup
Monday	Coco tea	Green juice	Vichyssoise	Green juice	Tomato and basil soup	Green juice	Pesto green soup
Tuesday	Lemon tea	Red juice	Cream of peas	Red juice	Green artichoke and bean soup	Red juice	Carrot, coriander and sesame seeds
Wednesday	Coco tea	Green juice	Purple cream	Green juice	Pesto green soup	Green juice	Tomato and basil soup
Thursday	Lemon tea	Red juice	Cucumber and grass	Red juice	Green garden lime soup	Red juice	Asian detox
Friday	Coco tea	Green juice	Avocado dream	Green juice	Popete chia soup	Green juice	Green garden lime soup
Saturday	Lemon tea	Red juice	Asparagus	Red juice	Asian detox	Red juice	Popeye chia soup

Sönd

For more information, go to: www.sondskin.com

Your Detox shopping list

The Staple Ingredients

These are your store cupboard staples. I advise buying the best quality you can find, in the quantity of your choice - often the larger the bottle, jar or packet, the better the value overall.

- Extra virgin olive oil
- Avocado oil
- Tahini
- Chia seeds
- Sesame seeds
- Pumpkin seeds
- Dried white beans
- Almond flakes
- Unsalted cashew nuts
- Unsalted, peeled almonds
- Ground almonds
- Fennel seeds
- Coriander seeds
- Dried cumin
- Dried thyme
- Salt (the best is Himalayan or Celtic sea salt)
- Black pepper
- Chilli powder
- Coconut milk

The Staple Herbs

I also advise buying all of your fresh herbs at this point too, then washing and chopping them and storing them immediately in the freezer wrapped in paper towels.

- Parsley
- Mint
- Dill
- Tarragon
- Thyme
- Chives
- Basil
- Lemongrass
- Coriander
- Celery leaves
- Bay leaves

Homemade Vegetable Stock

Vegetable stock is a staple part of soup making and is really easy to make in advance. I strongly advise making your own that can then be stored in the fridge and used throughout the week.

For 4.5L of vegetable stock:

- 5 onions
- 10 large carrots
- 5 fennel bulbs
- 3 large heads of celery
- 1 lemon
- 10 large tomatoes
- 5 courgettes
- 15 bay leaves
- 10g coriander seeds
- 10g fennel seeds
- 10g dried thyme
- 100g fresh parsley including stems
- 100g celery leaves
- Salt and black pepper to taste

See the previous chapter for how to make this amazing stock.

Your Detox shopping list

Days 1 to 4

These are the fresh ingredients you'll need for the first four days of your detox. I advise buying organic as much as you can.

- 7 lemons
- 2 large ginger roots
- 1 large turmeric root
- 2 vanilla pods
- 26 medium cucumbers
- 9 medium beetroots
- 10 bunches celery
- 22 medium carrots
- 6 green peppers
- 7 red peppers
- 27 tomatoes
- 8 large fennel bulbs
- 400g spinach
- 3 avocados
- 4 large onions
- 3 large leeks
- 3 large sweet potatoes
- 2 bunches spring onions
- 300g peas
- 4 parsnips
- 2 garlic bulbs
- 8 artichokes
- 100g lupin beans

Days 5 to 7

These are the fresh ingredients you'll need for the second half of your seven day detox. You'll notice that it's very similar to the first half, and if you have anything left over, feel free to use it. Fresh really is best so try to consume all of your fresh ingredients as soon as possible. Again, I advise buying organic as much as you can.

- 6 limes
- 6 lemons
- 2 large ginger roots
- 1 large turmeric root
- 1 vanilla pod
- 20 medium cucumbers
- 6 medium beetroots
- 10 bunches celery
- 16 medium carrots
- 6 red peppers
- 6 green peppers
- 12 tomatoes
- 400g spinach
- 2 avocados
- 3 large leeks
- 1 bunch spring onions
- 750g asparagus
- 1 garlic bulb
- 500g broccoli
- 240g green beans
- 360g courgette
- Red pepper

Alkaline Vegetable Stock
Your Nourishing Foundation

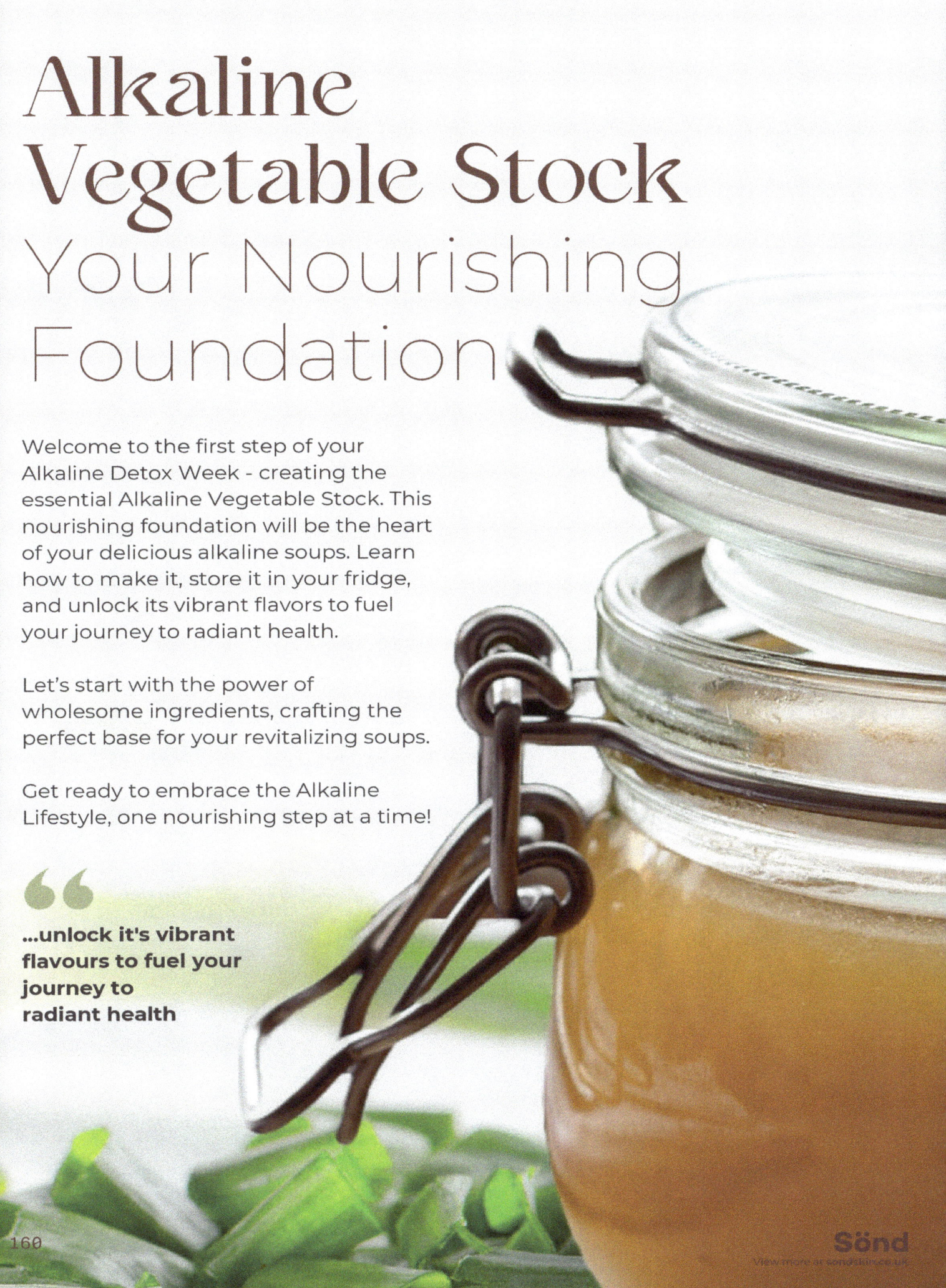

Welcome to the first step of your Alkaline Detox Week - creating the essential Alkaline Vegetable Stock. This nourishing foundation will be the heart of your delicious alkaline soups. Learn how to make it, store it in your fridge, and unlock its vibrant flavors to fuel your journey to radiant health.

Let's start with the power of wholesome ingredients, crafting the perfect base for your revitalizing soups.

Get ready to embrace the Alkaline Lifestyle, one nourishing step at a time!

> **...unlock it's vibrant flavours to fuel your journey to radiant health**

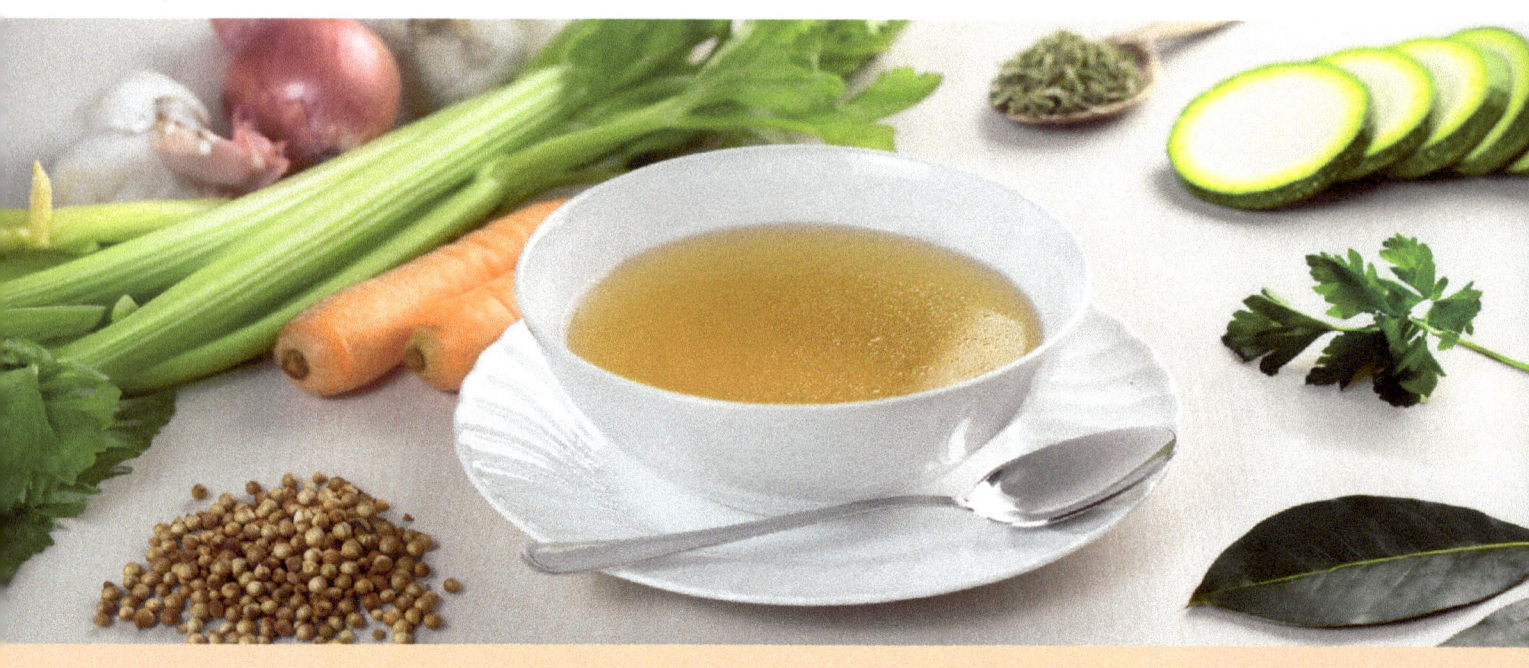

Alkaline Vegetable Stock

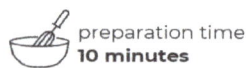 preparation time **10 minutes**  cooking time **10 minutes** 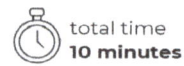 total time **10 minutes** 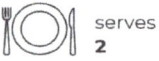 serves **2** 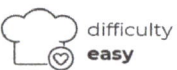 difficulty **easy**

INGREDIENTS

+ 1 large onion, peeled and cut in half
+ 2 large carrots, peeled and cut in half widthways
+ 1 fennel bulb, cut in half 3 large celery stalks
+ 1 slice of lemon
+ 2 large tomatoes, cut in half
+ 1 courgette, cut in half widthways
+ 3 bay leaves
+ 2g coriander seeds
+ 2g fennel seeds
+ 2g dried thyme
+ 20g fresh parsley including stems
+ 20g celery leaves
+ Salt and black pepper to taste

DIRECTIONS

1. Place all of the ingredients into a large saucepan and cover with 3L of cold water. Cover the pan and bring it to a boil.

2. Once boiling, reduce the heat and allow to simmer for 60 minutes.

3. Remove from the hob and allow to cool completely. Drain the stock through a colander, discard the solid vegetables and store in the fridge for up to seven days.

...unlock its vibrant flavors to fuel your journey to radiant health

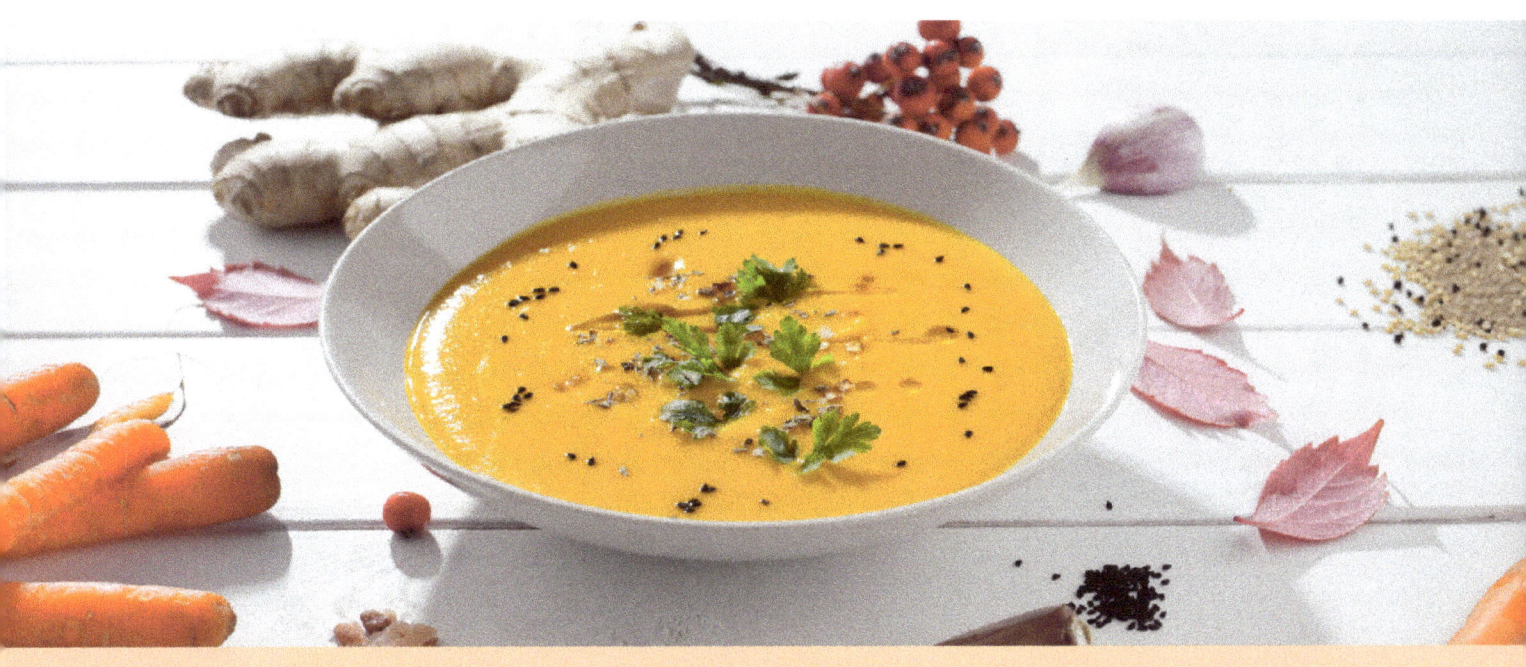

Carrot, Coriander & Sesame Seed Soup

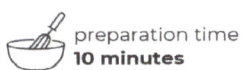 preparation time **10 minutes**    cooking time **20 minutes**   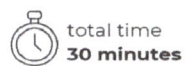 total time **30 minutes**    serves **2**   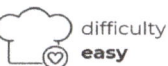 difficulty **easy**

INGREDIENTS

+ Extra virgin olive oil or avocado oil
+ 2 shallots, chopped
+ 1 large sweet potato, chopped
+ 2 cloves garlic, finely chopped
+ 1.5cm fresh ginger, peeled and grated
+ 1st Checklist item
+ 800ml vegetable stock
+ 250g fresh spinach leaves
+ 2 tbsp chia seeds (soaked in water for 20 min)
+ Salt and pepper
+ 1 tbsp sesamin seeds

DIRECTIONS

1. Heat the oil in a pan, add the shallots, sweet potato and garlic, cover and cook until tender.

2. Add the ginger and cook for one minute. Add the stock and bring to the boil until the sweet potato is cooked.

3. Remove from the heat, add the spinach and chia seeds and leave for 15 minutes.

4. Blend until smooth, add a drizzle of oil and salt and pepper and sprinkle with sesamin seeds.

Notes

You will need a blender for this recipe.

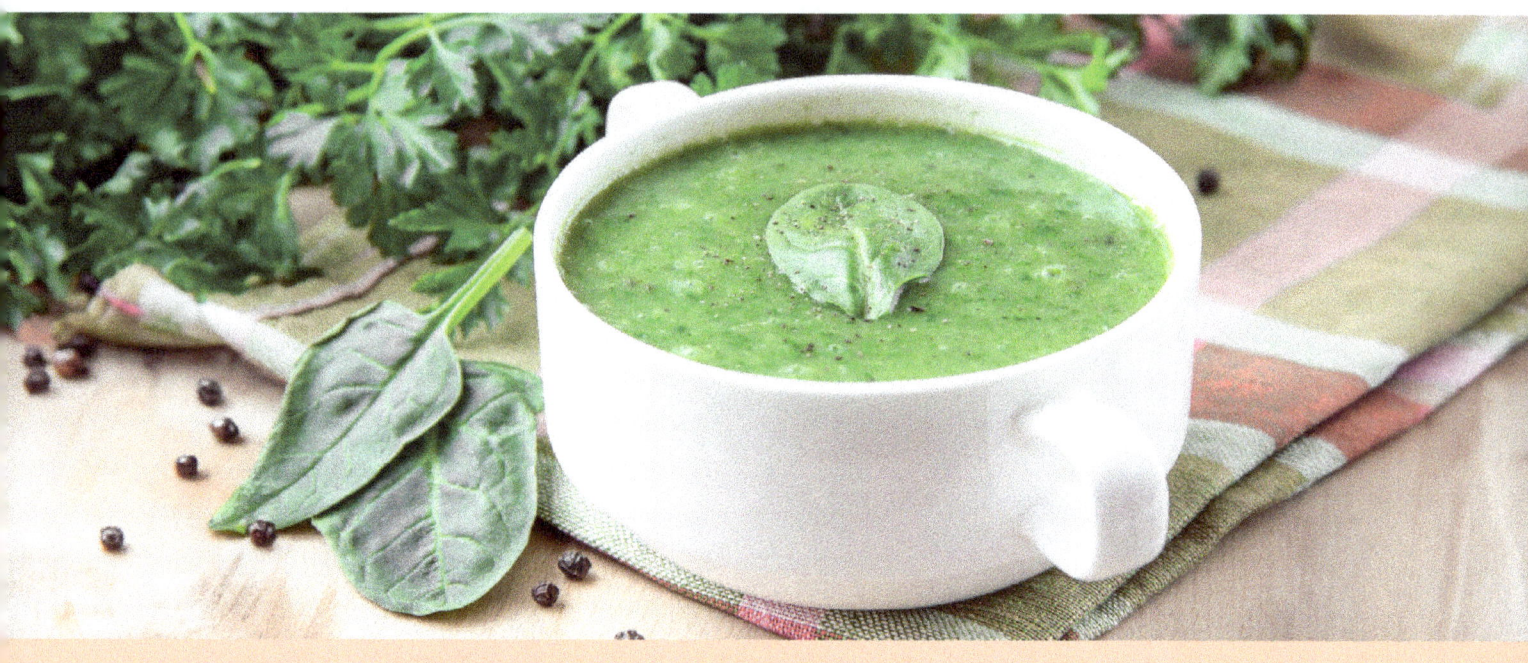

Popey Chia Soup

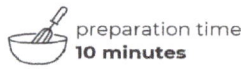 preparation time **10 minutes**
 cooking time **15 minutes**
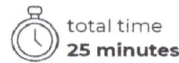 total time **25 minutes**
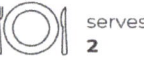 serves **2**
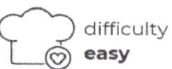 difficulty **easy**

INGREDIENTS

+ Extra virgin olive oil or avocado oil
+ 2 shallots, chopped
+ 1 large sweet potato, chopped
+ 2 cloves garlic, finely chopped
+ 1.5cm fresh ginger, peeled and grated
+ 800ml vegetable stock
+ 250g fresh spinach leaves
+ 2 tbsp chia seeds (soaked in water for 20 min)
+ Salt and pepper
+ 1 tbsp almond flakes

DIRECTIONS

1. Heat the oil in a pan, add the shallots, sweet potato and garlic, cover and cook until tender.

2. Add the ginger and cook for one minute. Add the stock and bring to the boil until the sweet potato is cooked.

3. Remove from the heat, add the spinach and chia seeds and leave for 15 minutes.

4. Blend until smooth, add a drizzle of oil and salt and pepper and sprinkle with almond flakes.

Notes

You will need a blender for this recipe.

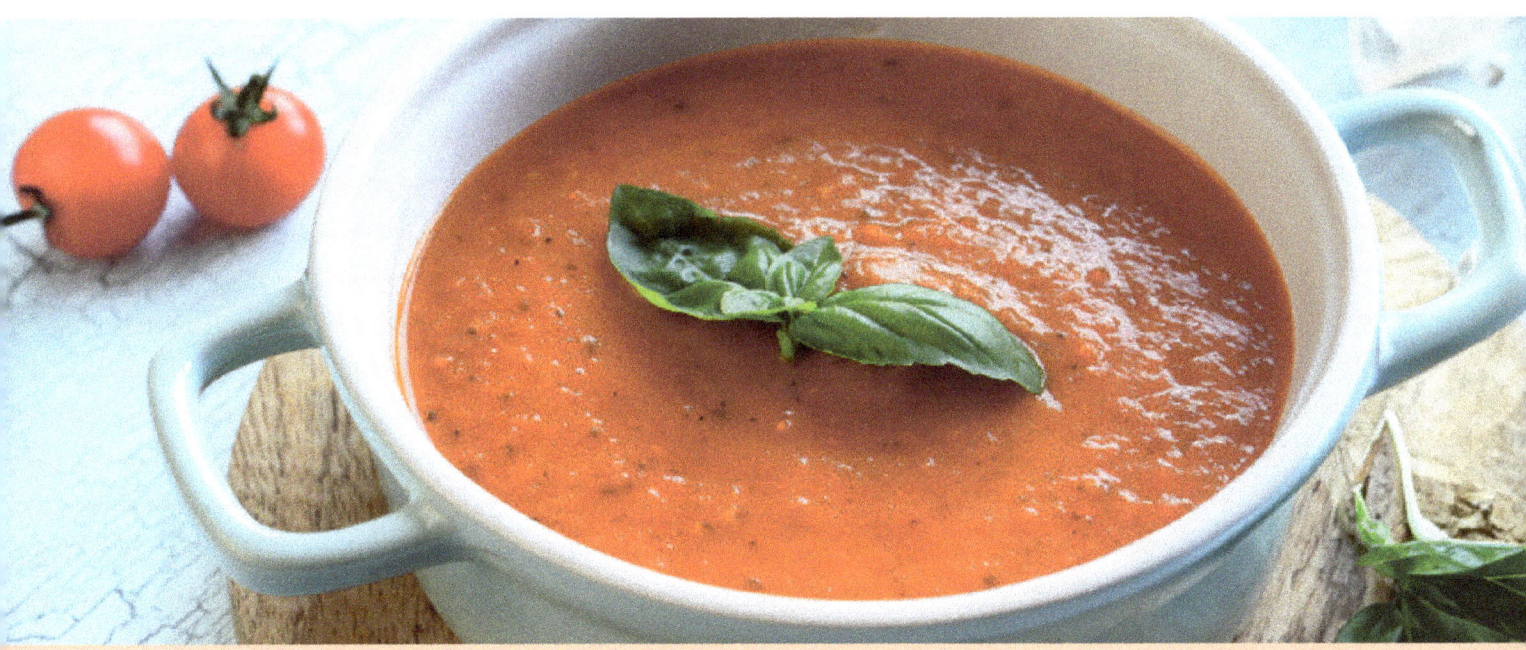

Tomato & Basil Soup

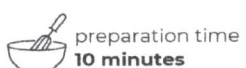 preparation time **10 minutes**
 cooking time **15 minutes**
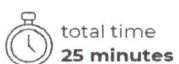 total time **25 minutes**
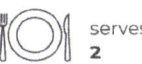 serves **2**
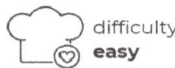 difficulty **easy**

INGREDIENTS

+ Extra virgin olive oil or avocado oil
+ 1 medium onion, chopped
+ 20g fresh basil with finely chopped stalks
+ 2 cloves garlic
+ 2 parsnips, peeled and chopped
+ 750g tomatoes, peeled and chopped
+ 750ml vegetable stock
+ 1 tbsp chia seeds (soaked in water for 20 minutes)
+ 1 tbsp pumpkin seeds
+ Salt and pepper
+ Chilli (optional)

DIRECTIONS

1. Heat the oil in a pan, add the onions, basil stalks and garlic, cover and cook until tender.

2. Add the parsnips, tomatoes and stock and bring to the boil until the parsnips are cooked.

3. Add the basil leaves, blend until smooth, add a drizzle of oil and salt and pepper and sprinkle with chia and pumpkin seeds and add chilli.

4. Heat the oil in a pan, add the asparagus, parsley and chives, add a splash of water and simmer until tender.

Notes

You will need a blender for this recipe.

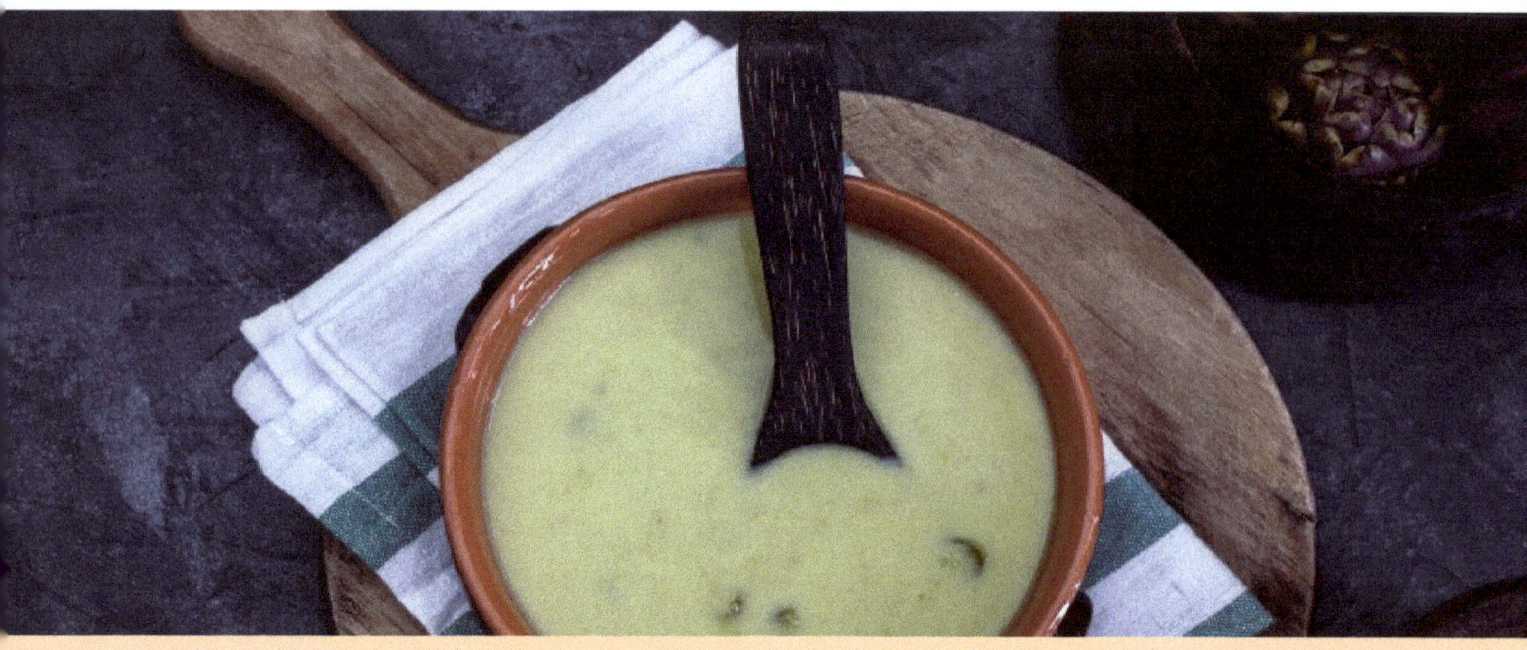

Green Artichoke & Bean Soup

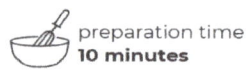 preparation time **10 minutes**    cooking time **25 minutes**   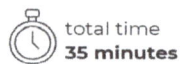 total time **35 minutes**   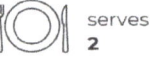 serves **2**   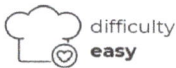 difficulty **easy**

INGREDIENTS

+ Extra virgin olive oil or avocado oil
+ 1 medium onion, chopped
+ 2 cloves garlic, finely chopped
+ 400g fresh white beans (soaked in water for 12-16 hours before cooking)
+ 4 artichokes, cleaned cut into spikes
+ 150g fresh tomatoes, skinned and chopped
+ Juice of 1 lemon
+ Bunch freshly chopped basil
+ 700ml vegetable stock
+ Salt and pepper
+ Chilli (optional)

DIRECTIONS

1. Heat the oil in a pan, add the onions and garlic, cover and cook until tender.

2. Add the beans, artichokes, tomatoes, lemon, basil and stock and bring to the boil for around 25 minutes.

3. Blend until smooth, add a drizzle of oil and salt and pepper and sprinkle with chilli.

Notes

You will need a blender for this recipe.

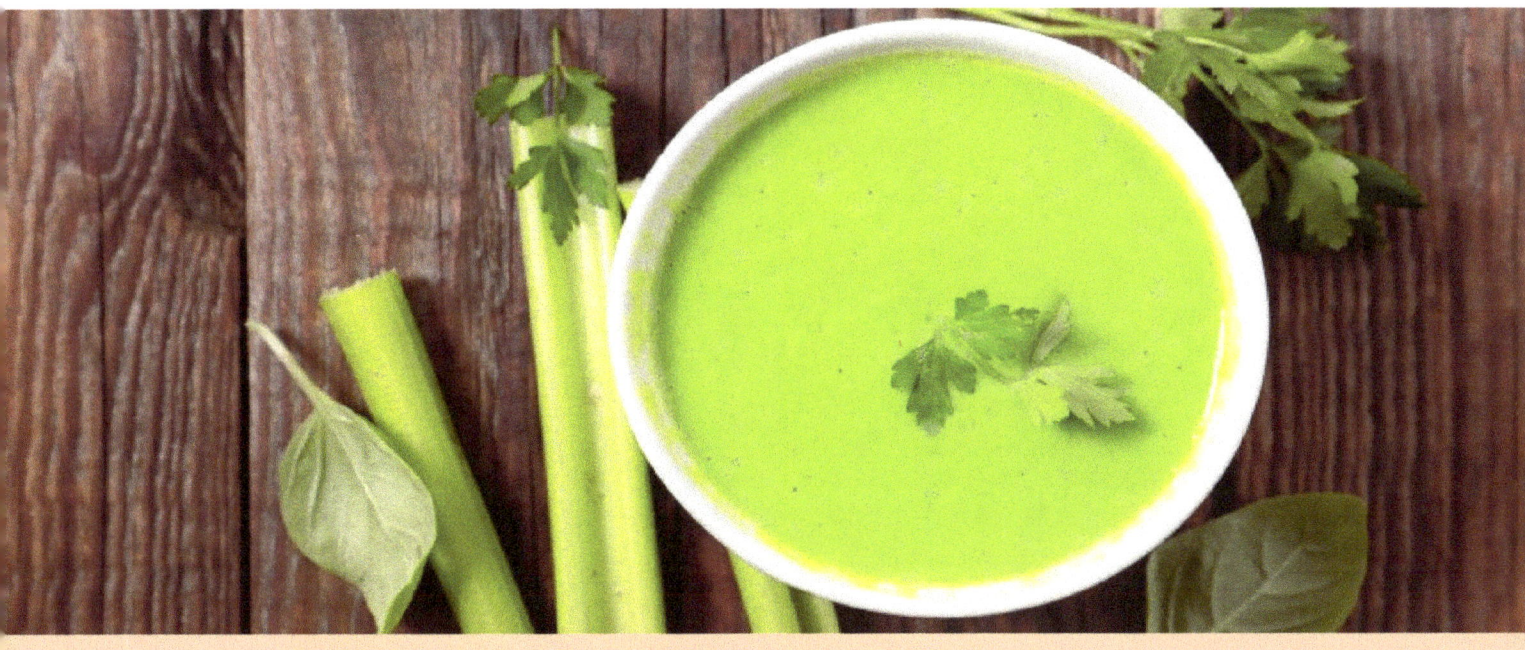

Pesto Green Soup

preparation time **10 minutes** cooking time **10 minutes** total time **20 minutes** serves **2** difficulty **easy**

INGREDIENTS

+ 50g fresh basil
+ 2 cloves of garlic
+ Salt and pepper
+ 30g ground almonds
+ 3-4 tablespoons olive oil
+ Pinch of chilli powder (optional)

DIRECTIONS

1. In a blender, mix the basil with the garlic, salt, pepper, ground almonds and olive oil until creamy.

2. Add chilli to taste.

INGREDIENTS

+ Extra virgin olive oil or avocado oil
+ 1 medium leek cut into half rounds
+ 4 stalks celery, chopped
+ 2 medium carrots, chopped
+ Small handful of fresh thyme
+ 180g courgettes, chopped
+ 700ml vegetable stock
+ Handful of fresh parsley
+ Salt and pepper

DIRECTIONS

1. Heat the oil in a pan, add the leeks, celery and carrots, cover and cook until tender.

2. Add the thyme and cook for two minutes.

3. Add the courgettes and cook for a further five minutes.

4. Add the stock and parsley and bring to the boil until the vegetables are just firm.

5. Blend until smooth, add a drizzle of oil and salt and pepper and drizzle with pesto.

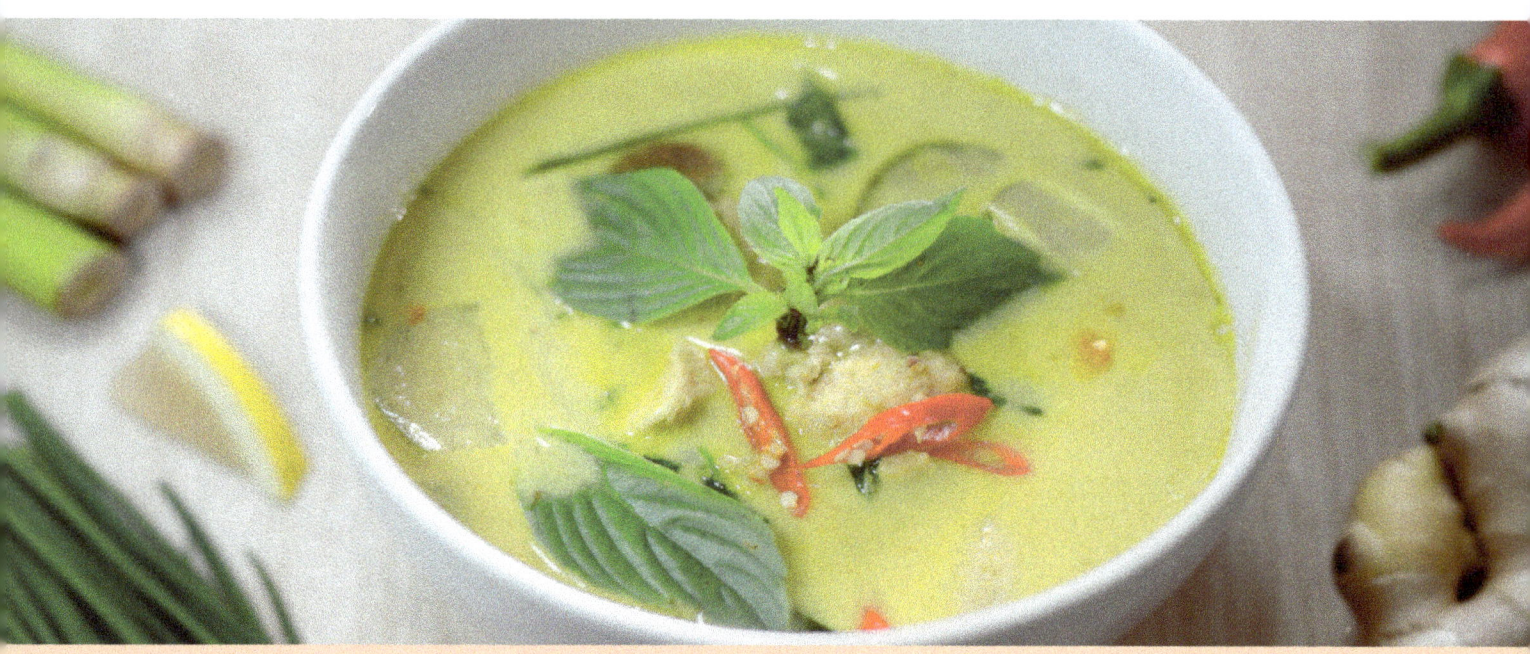

Asian Detox Soup

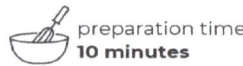 preparation time **10 minutes**
 cooking time **15 minutes**
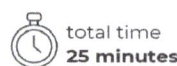 total time **25 minutes**
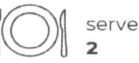 serves **2**
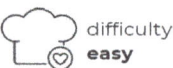 difficulty **easy**

INGREDIENTS

+ 400ml vegetable stock
+ Handful of fresh lemongrass cut lengthways
+ Handful of fresh chives
+ 3 spring onions, chopped
+ 1cm fresh ginger, peeled and grated
+ ½ red chilli pepper, sliced
+ Juice of 1 small lemon
+ 1 tsp grated lemon peel
+ Handful of fresh coriander
+ Handful of fresh parsley
+ 200ml coco milk

DIRECTIONS

1. Bring the stock to the boil and add all of the ingredients, except the coriander and parsley.

2. Cook over a low heat for 15 minutes. Add the coriander and parsley.

3. Remove from the heat and blend with the coco milk.

Notes

You will need a blender for this recipe.

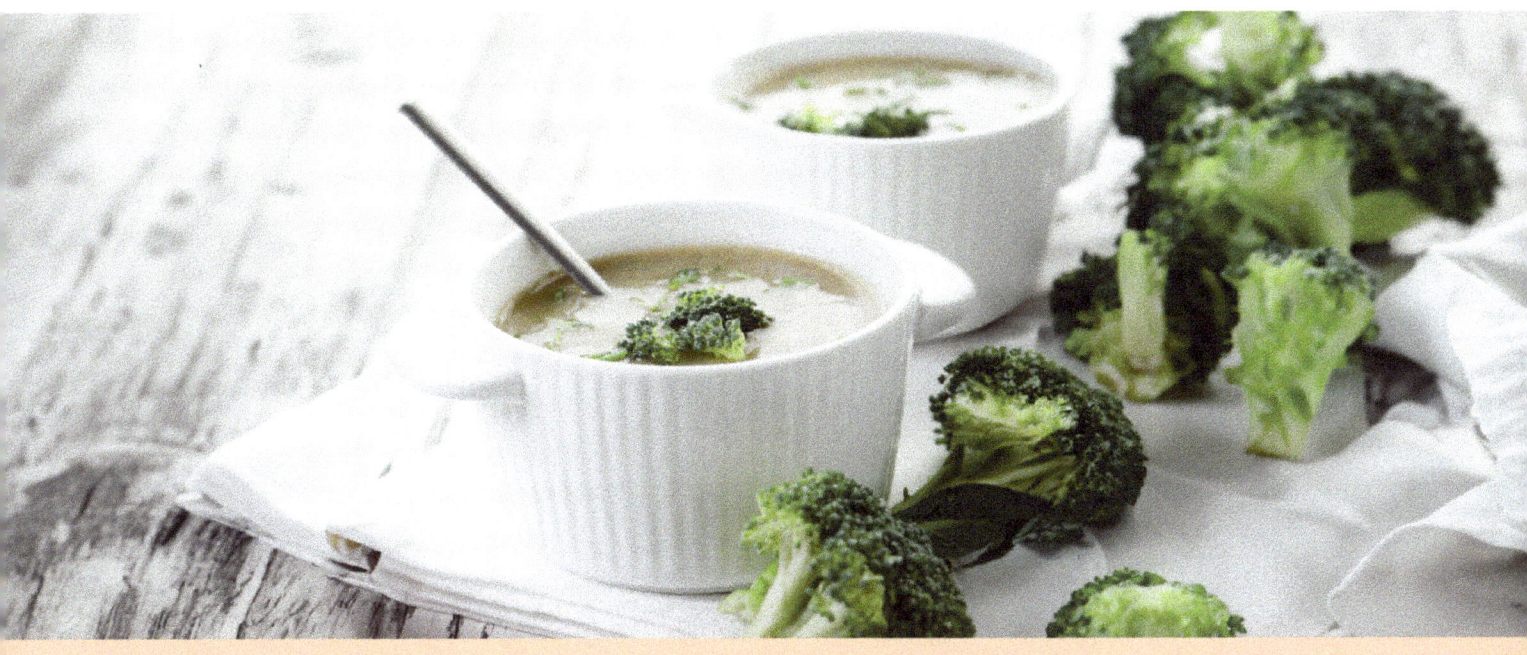

Green Garden Lime Soup

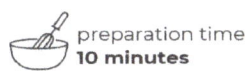 preparation time **10 minutes**  cooking time **15 minutes** 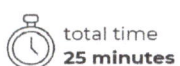 total time **25 minutes**  serves **2** 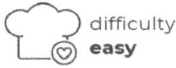 difficulty **easy**

INGREDIENTS

+ Extra virgin olive oil or avocado oil
+ 1 large shallot, chopped
+ 250g broccoli (chopped stalks and flowers divided into small florets)
+ 120g green beans, stringless and chopped
+ 150g asparagus, bases removed and chopped
+ Juice of 1 lime
+ 1.5cm fresh ginger, peeled and grated
+ 2 tbsp dill
+ 600ml vegetable stock
+ Salt and pepper
+ 1 tbsp cashew nuts

DIRECTIONS

1. Heat the oil in a pan, add the shallots, cover and cook until tender.

2. Add the broccoli stalks and cook for five minutes. Add the green beans and cook for a further five minutes.

3. Add the asparagus, broccoli florets, lime juice, ginger and dill.

4. Add the stock and bring to the boil until the vegetables are just firm.

5. Blend until smooth, add a drizzle of oil and salt and pepper and sprinkle with cashews.

Notes

You will need a blender for this recipe.

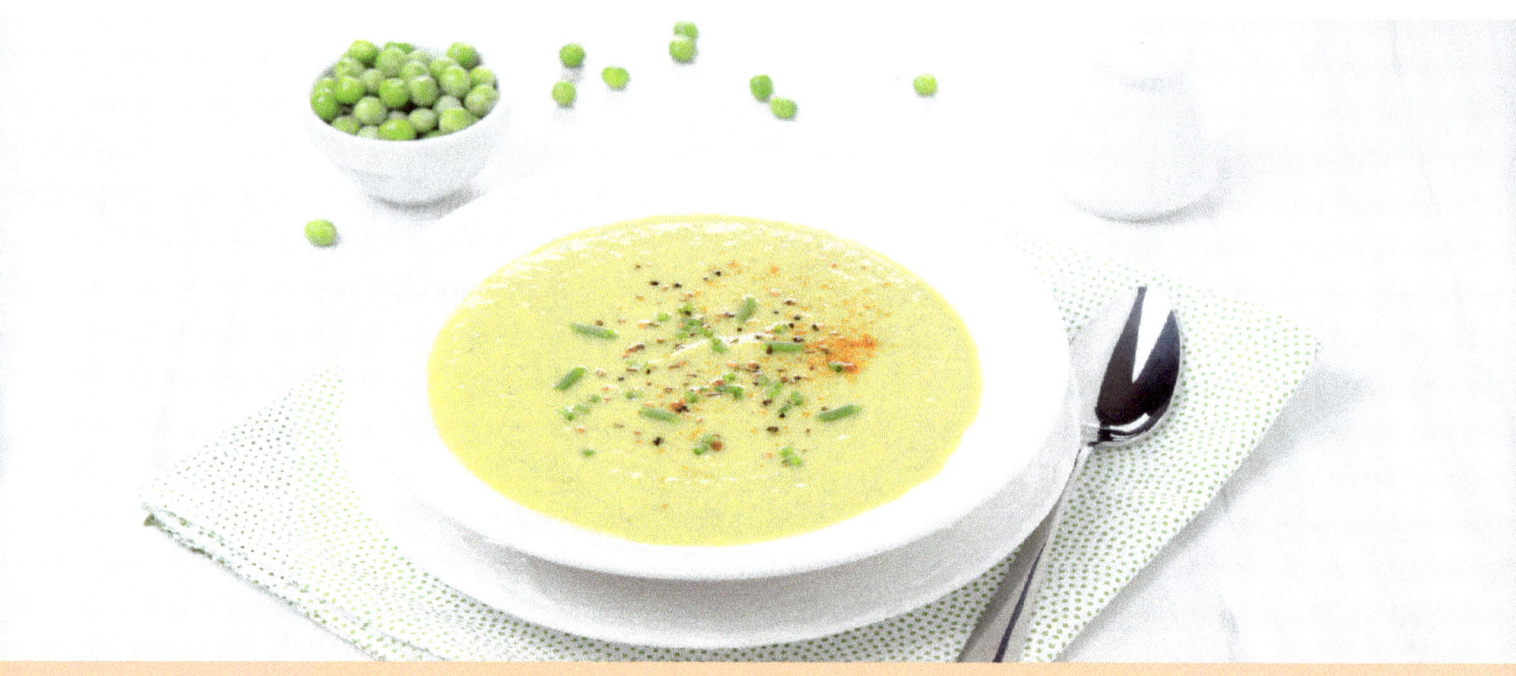

Cream of Peas Cold Soup

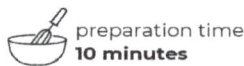 preparation time **10 minutes**  cooking time **10 minutes** 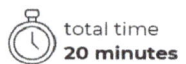 total time **20 minutes** 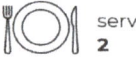 serves **2** 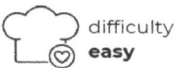 difficulty **easy**

INGREDIENTS

+ Extra virgin olive oil or avocado oil
+ 500ml water
+ 300g peas
+ 1/2 fennel, chopped
+ Handful of fresh tarragon
+ Handful of fresh parsley
+ Salt and pepper
+ Fennel seeds (optional)

DIRECTIONS

1. Heat the oil in a pan, add the peas and fennel, add some water and simmer for three minutes.

2. Add the tarragon and parsley and blend until smooth.

3. Pour in the rest of the water and bring to the boil.

4. Add salt and pepper and sprinkle with fennel seeds if you like.

Notes

You will need a blender for this recipe.

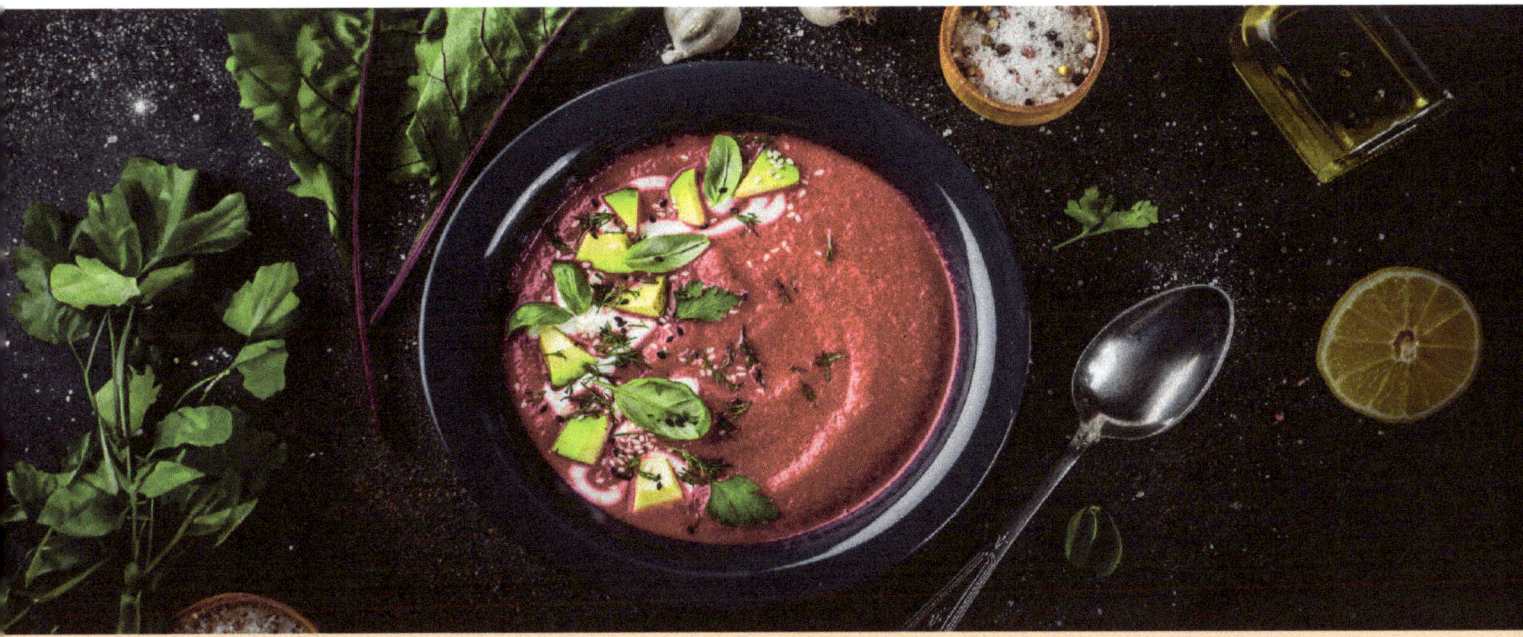

Purple Cream Cold Soup

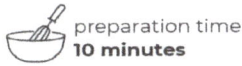 preparation time **10 minutes**    cooking time **15 minutes**   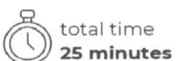 total time **25 minutes**   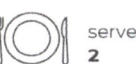 serves **2**   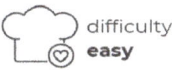 difficulty **easy**

INGREDIENTS

+ Extra virgin olive oil or avocado oil
+ 2 carrots, chopped
+ 500ml water
+ 350g beetroot, peeled and chopped
+ ½ fennel, chopped
+ Handful of fresh thyme
+ Handful of fresh parsley
+ Salt and pepper
+ Fennel seeds (optional)

DIRECTIONS

1. Heat the oil in a pan, add the carrots, cover and cook for 15 minutes or until tender.

2. Pour in the water and bring to the boil.

3. Add the beetroot and fennel and simmer for three minutes.

4. Add the thyme and parsley and blend until smooth.

5. Add salt and pepper and sprinkle with fennel seeds.

Notes

You will need a blender for this recipe.

Sönd
View more at **sondskin.co.uk**

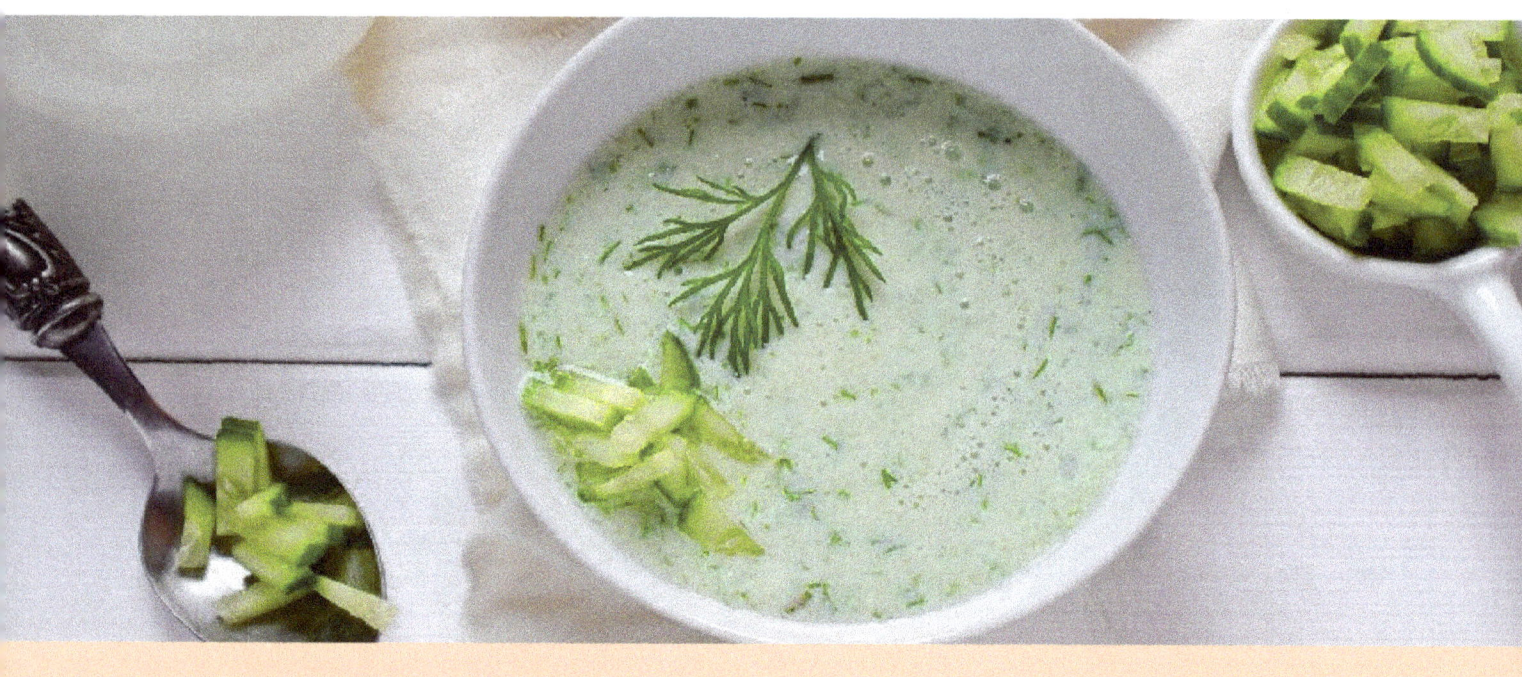

Cucumber & Grass Cold Soup

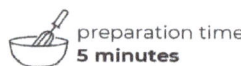 preparation time **5 minutes**
 cooking time **5 minutes**
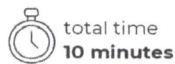 total time **10 minutes**
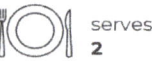 serves **2**
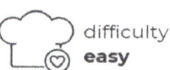 difficulty **easy**

INGREDIENTS

+ 2 cucumbers, chopped
+ 1 avocado, peeled and cut into large chunks
+ Juice of 2 limes
+ Handful of fresh dill
+ Handful of fresh mint
+ Salt and pepper

DIRECTIONS

1. Blend all of the ingredients until smooth and season with salt and pepper.

Notes

You will need a blender for this recipe.

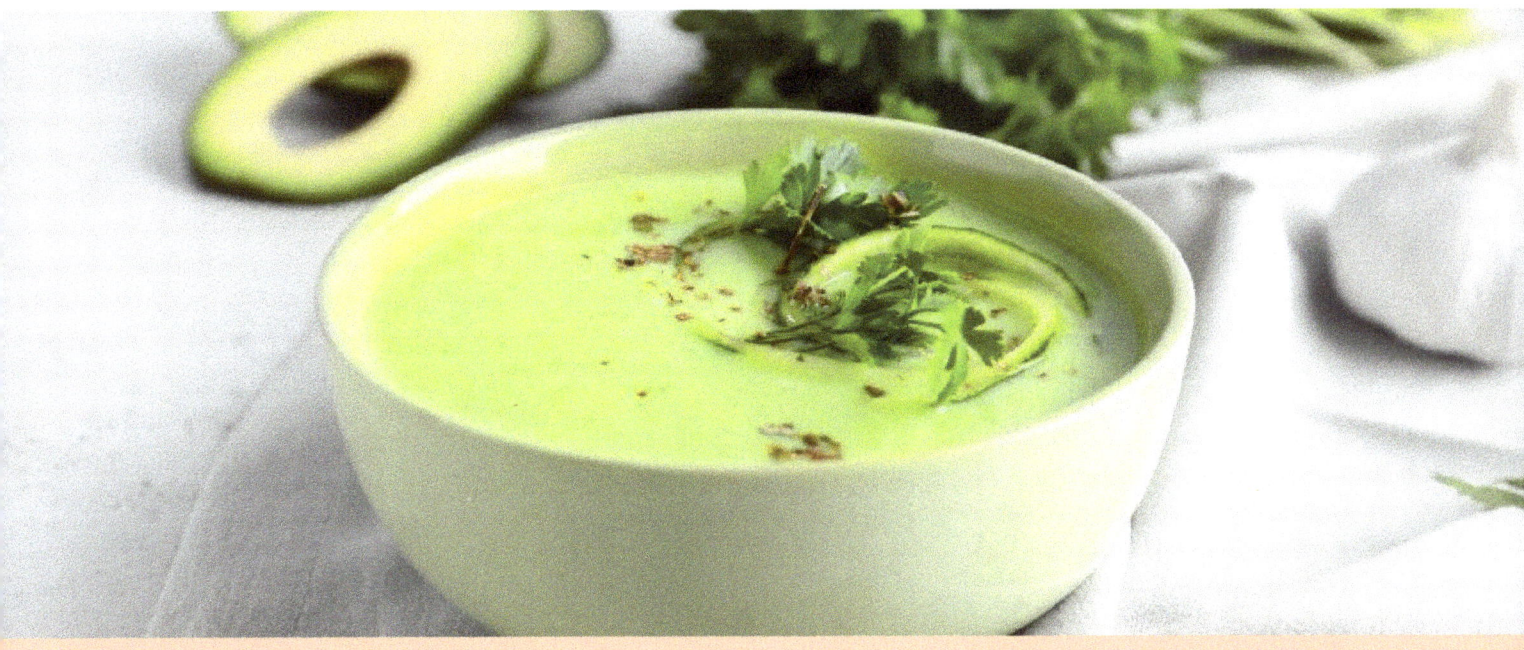

Avocado Dream Cold Soup

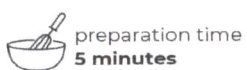 preparation time **5 minutes**  cooking time **5 minutes** 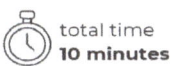 total time **10 minutes** 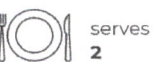 serves **2** 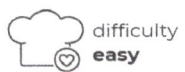 difficulty **easy**

INGREDIENTS

+ 1 avocado, peeled and cut into large chunks
+ 100g precooked lupins
+ Handful of fresh parsley
+ Pinch of fresh chives
+ 200 ml water
+ Juice of 2 limes
+ Olive or avocado oil
+ Salt and pepper

DIRECTIONS

1. Blend all of the ingredients except the oil until smooth. Season and drizzle with oil.

Notes

You will need a blender for this recipe.

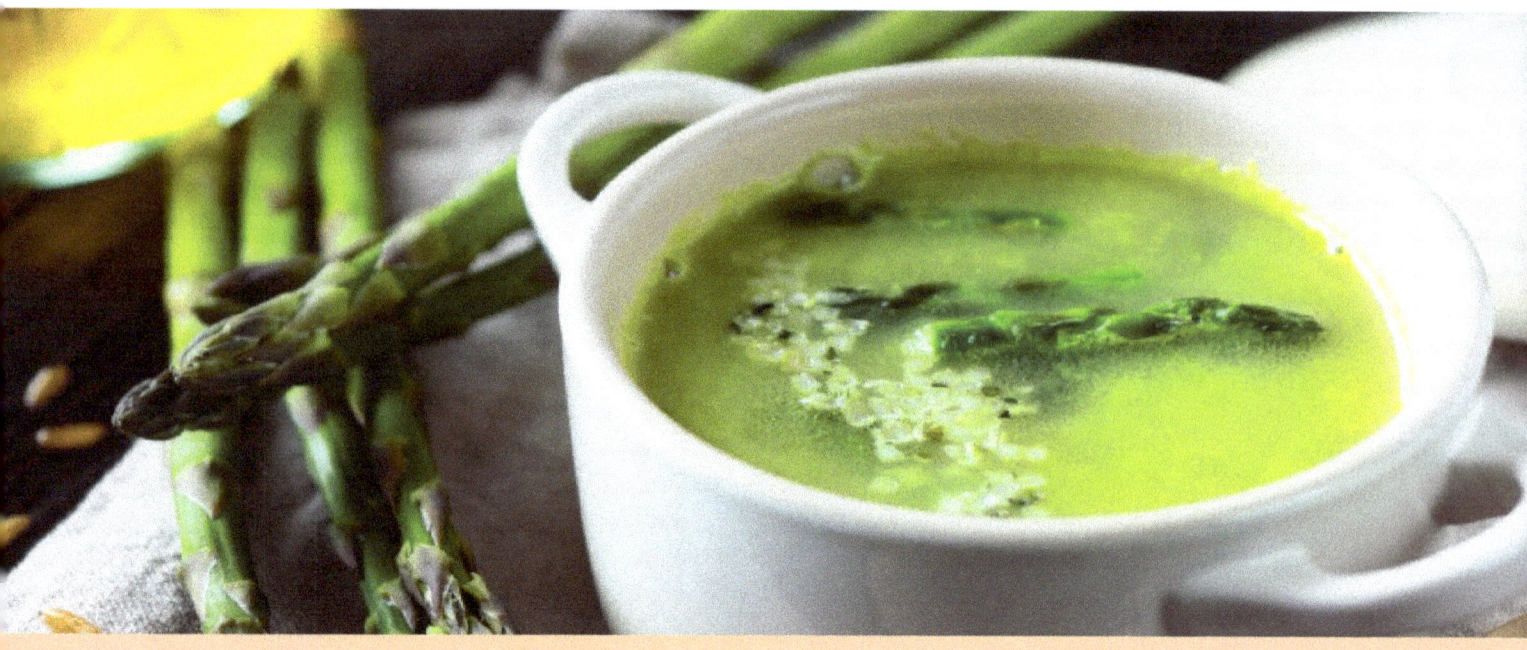

Asparagus Cold Soup

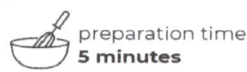 preparation time **5 minutes**  cooking time **10 minutes** 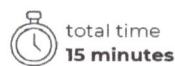 total time **15 minutes** 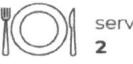 serves **2** 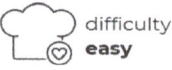 difficulty **easy**

INGREDIENTS

+ Extra virgin olive oil or avocado oil
+ 400ml water
+ 450g asparagus, base removed and chopped
+ Handful of fresh parsley
+ Pinch of fresh chives
+ Juice of 2 limes
+ Olive oil or avocado oil
+ Salt and pepper
+ Almonds or cashews (optional)

DIRECTIONS

1. Heat the oil in a pan, add the asparagus, parsley and chives, add a splash of water and simmer until tender.

2. Pour in the rest of the water and bring to the boil.

3. Add the lime juice, blend until smooth, add a drizzle of oil and salt and pepper and sprinkle with almonds or cashews.

Notes

You will need a blender for this recipe.

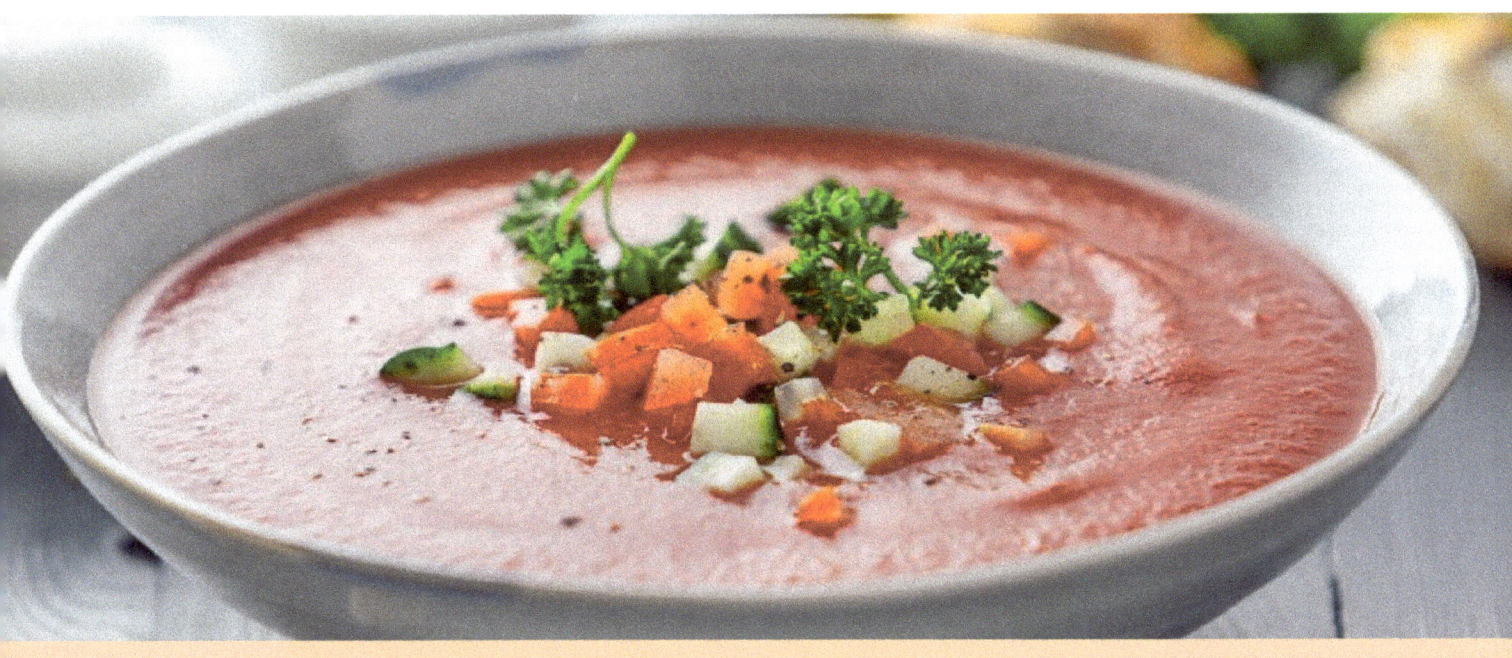

Gazpacho

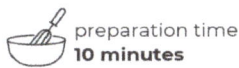 preparation time **10 minutes**
 cooking time **5 minutes**
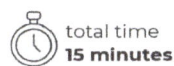 total time **15 minutes**
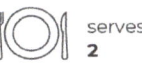 serves **2**
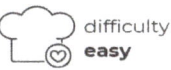 difficulty **easy**

INGREDIENTS

+ 250g tomatoes, chopped
+ 1/2 avocado
+ 1 red pepper, seeds removed, chopped
+ 150g cucumber, chopped
+ 2 tsp extra virgin olive oil or avocado oil
+ Bunch of fresh parsley
+ Bunch of fresh basil
+ Pinch salt and pepper
+ Pumpkin seeds, sesame seeds, almonds or cashews (optional)

DIRECTIONS

1. Blend the ingredients in a high powered blender, saving the cucumber and avocado until near the end, until you achieve a smooth consistency.

2. Season to taste and add a drizzle of olive or avocado oil before serving.

3. Add a sprinkling of pumpkin or sesame seeds, almonds or cashews.

Notes

You will need a blender for this recipe.

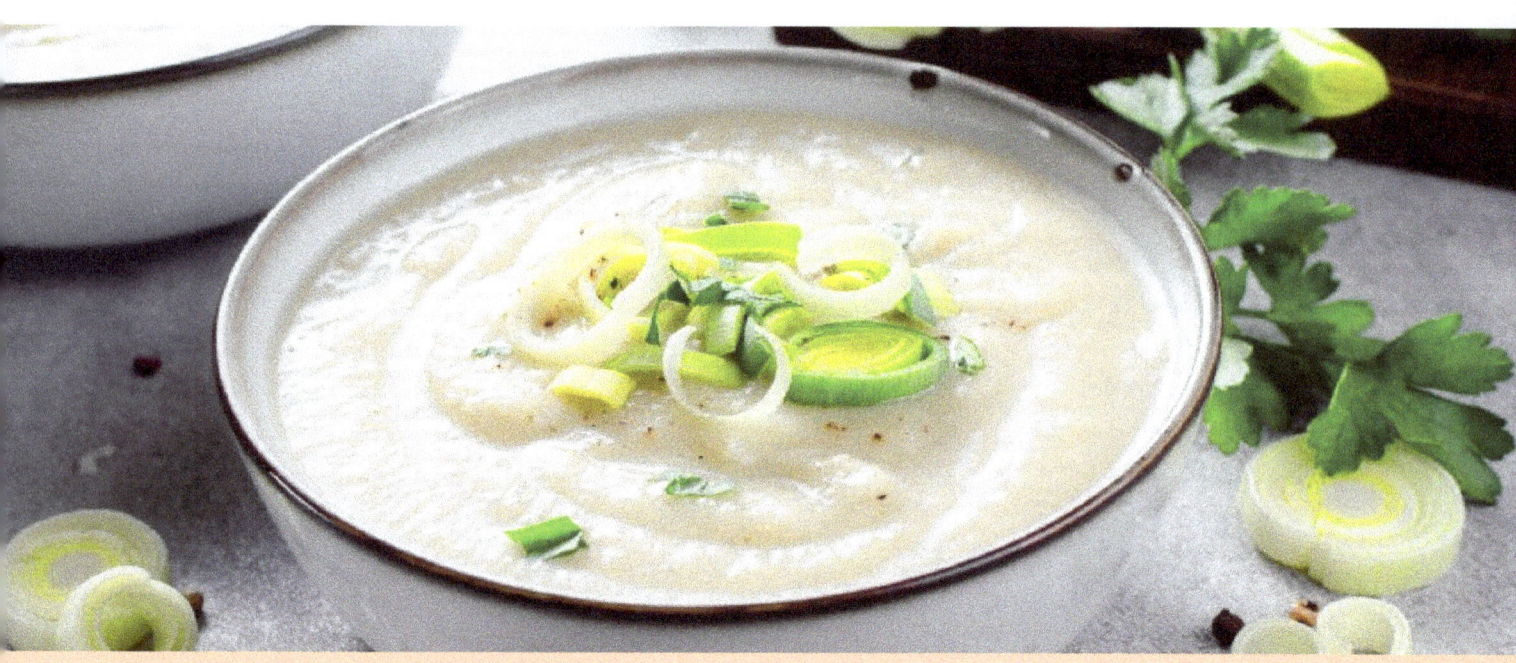

Vichyssoise

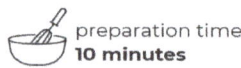 preparation time **10 minutes**    cooking time **20 minutes**   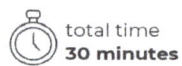 total time **30 minutes**   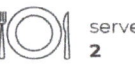 serves **2**   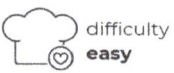 difficulty **easy**

INGREDIENTS

+ Extra virgin olive oil or avocado oil
+ 1 sweet potato, chopped, cooked in boiling water
+ 1 fennel finely chopped
+ 500ml water
+ Bunch of fresh dill
+ Bunch of fresh parsley
+ Salt and pepper
+ Pumpkin seeds, sesame seeds, almonds or cashews (optional)

DIRECTIONS

1. Heat the oil in a pan, add the sweet potato and fennel, cover and cook for ten minutes stirring occasionally.

2. When the vegetables have coloured, add the water, bring to the boil and simmer for 20 minutes.

3. Add the dill and parsley and blend until smooth.

4. Add a drizzle of oil and salt and pepper and a sprinkling of seeds, almonds or cashews.

Notes

You will need a blender for this recipe.

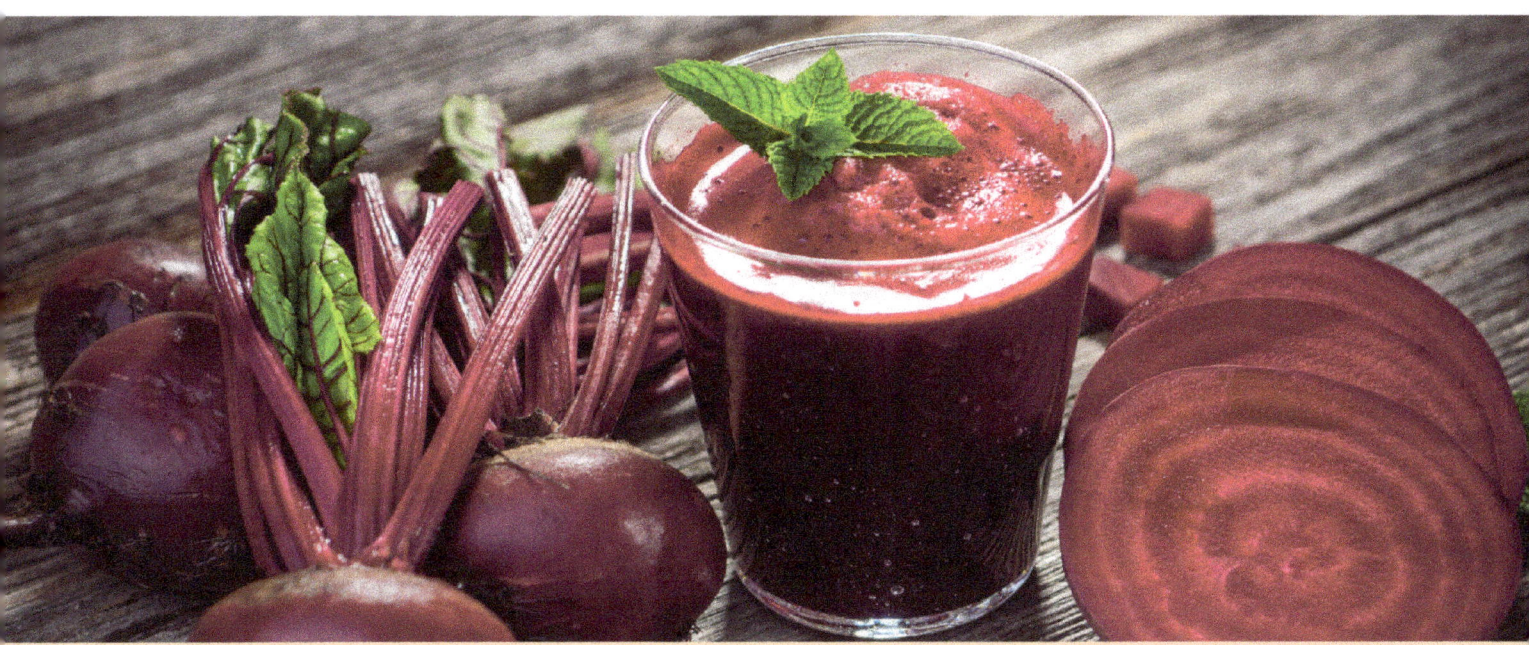

Red Juice

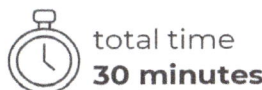 total time **30 minutes**

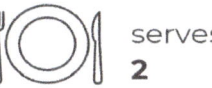 serves **2**

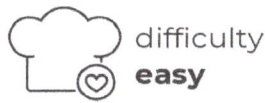 difficulty **easy**

INGREDIENTS

+ 2 large cucumbers
+ 1cm whole ginger, peeled and grated
+ 1 large beetroot
+ 4 stalks of celery plus leaves
+ 2 large carrots
+ 1 large red pepper
+ 2 tomatoes
+ 2 tbsp chia seeds

DIRECTIONS

1. Add all of the vegetables to a juicer or extractor and create a juice.

2. Stir in the chia seeds at the end.

Notes

You will need a slow speed extractor for this recipe.

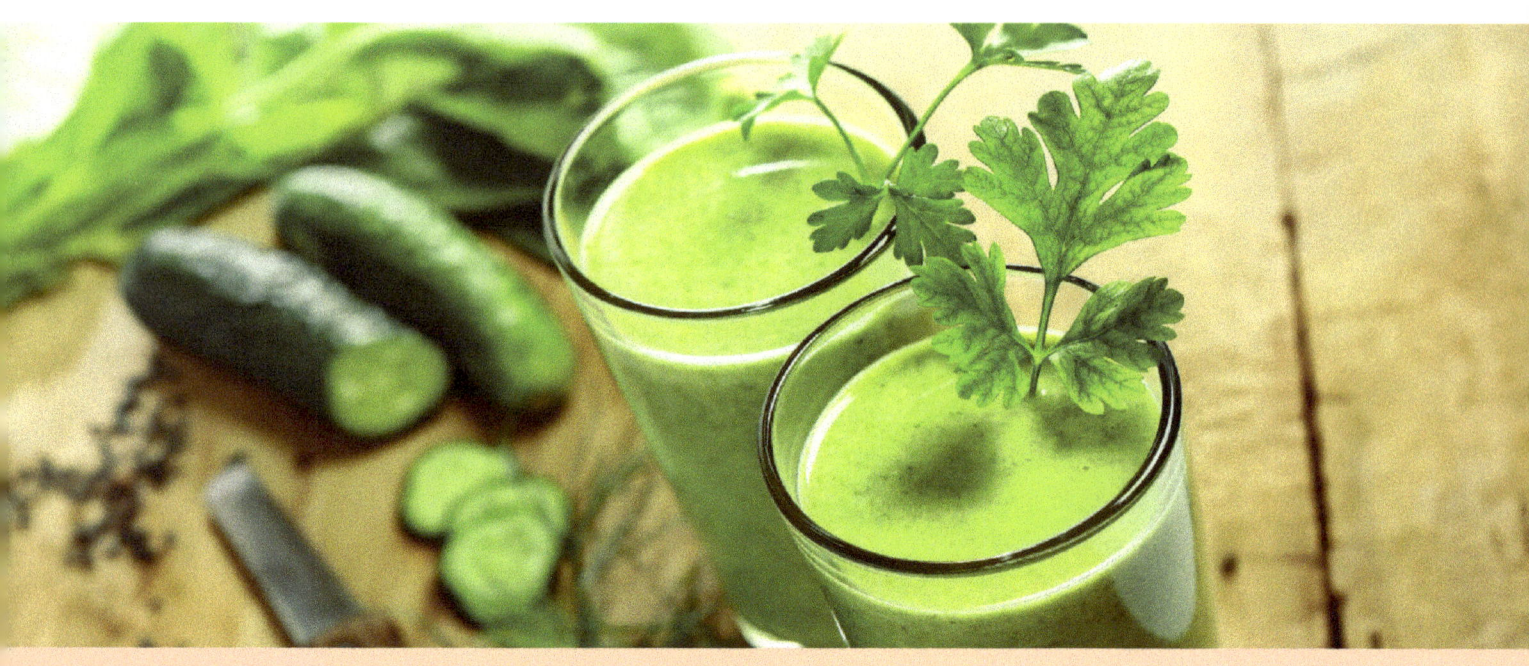

Green Juice

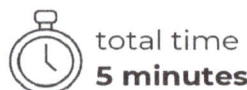 total time
5 minutes

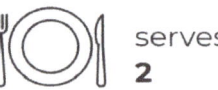 serves
2

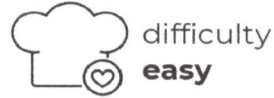 difficulty
easy

INGREDIENTS

+ 2 large cucumbers
+ 1cm whole ginger, peeled and grated
+ 6 stalks of celery plus leaves
+ Large bunch fresh parsley
+ Large bunch fresh mint
+ 1 large fennel
+ 1 large green pepper
+ 4 handfuls of spinach
+ Squeeze of fresh lemon

DIRECTIONS

1. Add all of the vegetables to a juicer or extractor and create a juice.

2. Stir in the chia seeds at the end.

Notes

You will need a slow speed extractor for this recipe.

Sönd
View more at **sondskin.co.uk**

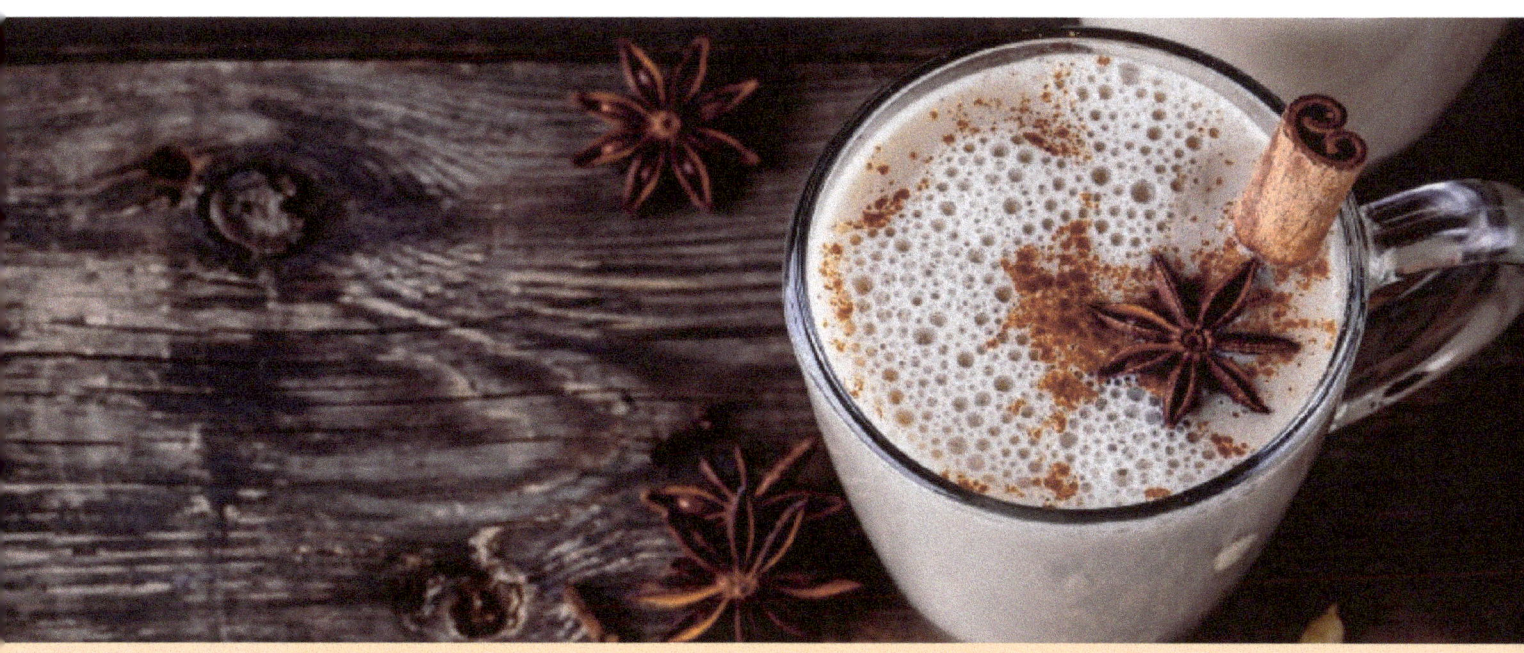

Coco Tea

 total time **5 minutes**

 serves **1**

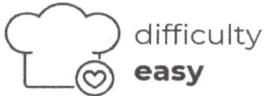 difficulty **easy**

DIRECTIONS

+ Add 1cm of whole ginger, peeled and grated, to a mug
+ Add one cinnamon pod Pour on warmed coconut milk
+ Add a sprinkling of turmeric (optional) Strain and enjoy

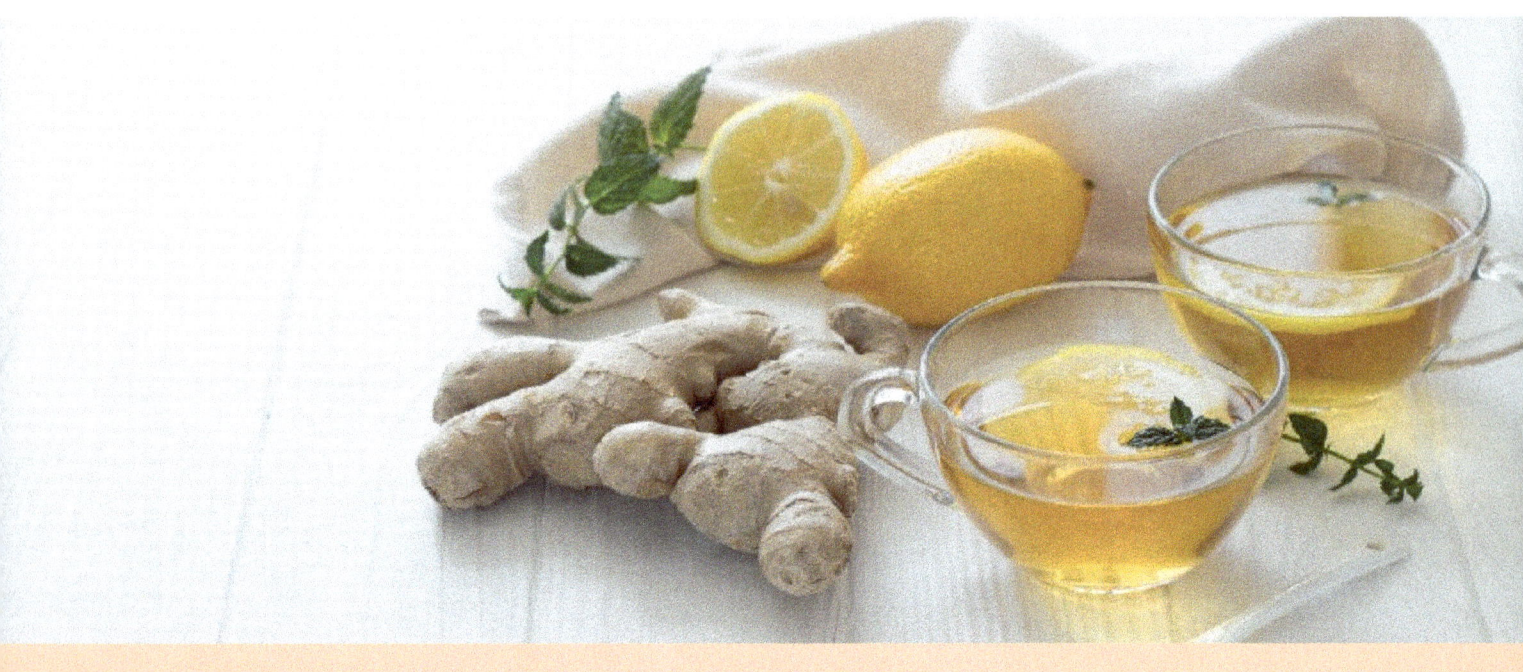

Lemon Tea

 total time
5 minutes

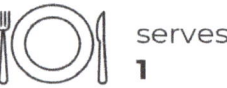 serves
1

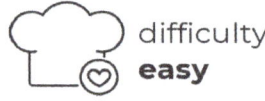 difficulty
easy

DIRECTIONS

+ Add the juice of one lemon to a mug
+ Add 1cm of whole ginger, peeled and grated
+ Pour on boiling water and leave to steep for five minutes
+ Add a sprinkling of turmeric (optional)
+ Strain and enjoy

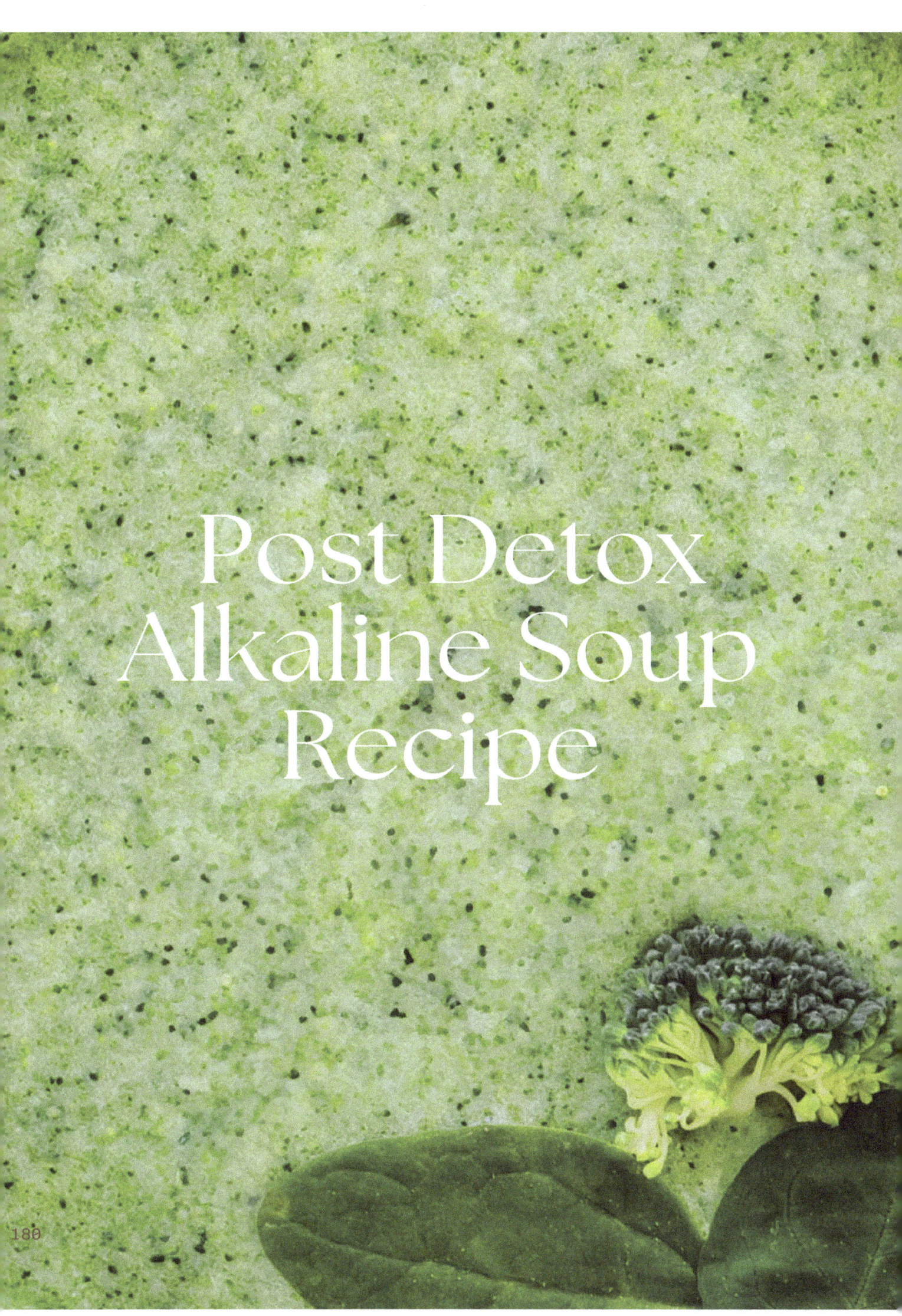

Post Detox Alkaline Soup Recipe

How to make a soup

As you've more than likely noticed, soups make up the huge majority of the foods included in my seven day alkalising detox. But they also make up an important part of the everyday alkaline lifestyle.

I've included all the necessary ingredients and recipes for each soup in the detox chapters, but I thought it would be helpful to talk about the basics of soup making, for after your detox and as you embrace your new alkaline lifestyle.

Each soup will use your vegetable stock, so make sure you've always got a batch to hand. All soup making tends to follow the same basic rules...

> **a journey that revitalizes your body and rejuvenates your spirit.**

RULE 1.
Base
The basics of any soup are an ingredient from the onion family (either onion, leeks or spring onion) plus carrots and celery. They all need to be chopped into small pieces and then lightly fried in extra virgin olive or avocado oil.

RULE 2.
Herbs and Spices
Herbs and spices enhance the flavour of any dish, and can be used fresh or dried. Add herbs and spices to the fried onions, carrots and celery, and only ever let them cook in a dry pan for less than a minute.

RULE 3.
Thickeners and Protein
Soups can be thickened by adding sweet potato, beans, lentils, quinoa and other seed grains mentioned in my alkaline food list further on in this book. I don't use too many thickeners in the seven day detox, but feel free to introduce more after your detox as you embrace your alkaline lifestyle.

Sönd
View more at sondskin.co.uk

RULE 4.
Combining Vegetables
Each individual soup tends to have one main vegetable which is then combined with other alkaline vegetables. Each vegetable should be added one at a time, each one cooked for 1 to 2 minutes before the next is added, depending on cooking time. I tend to group vegetables together in soups, such as green vegetables for a colourful green soup, fennel or liquorice for intense flavour or carrots, parsnips and sweet potatoes for sweetness. After your seven day detox, you can add vegetables from the acid-forming list if you like, remembering to stick to the 80:20 rule (80% alkaline, 20% acid-forming).

RULE 5.
Time for Stock
Add as much vegetable stock as a recipe suggests or adjust to your personal tastes. Add more for a thinner soup, add less if you prefer a thicker soup.

RULE 6.
Consistency
In my detox soup recipes, I've recommended blending each soup, using either a soup maker or stick blender. It's really a personal choice whether you prefer a smooth soup or a more rustic soup with more consistency. During your detox I recommend blending each soup to stick to the liquid theme, but when you're living your alkaline lifestyle, you can choose. I tend to suggest blended soups at lunchtime as they're easier to eat if you're pushed for time. In the evening you can opt for a rustic soup that contains vegetable pieces - chewing makes us feel fuller, and therefore we're likely to consume a smaller portion. This is useful in order to not overburden our digestive systems in the evening before bed to reduce the digestive processes that will need to occur overnight, risking an increase of acidity in the body.

RULE 7.
Making Soups More Filling
As long as you always keep in mind the 80:20 rule, you can use a soup as a base for a complete meal by adding gluten free pasta, meat, fish or seafood. Plant-based protein-rich foods such as beans, lentils and chickpeas are also ideal. However, they need careful planning - soak all dried beans, pulses and legumes in water overnight and cook according to the packet instructions before adding to your soups.

RULE 8.
The Final Touch
All soups can be enhanced with a little extra such as a drizzle of olive oil and salt and pepper to taste. You can then also add seeds, almond flames, cashew nuts or chopped avocado for texture.

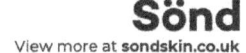

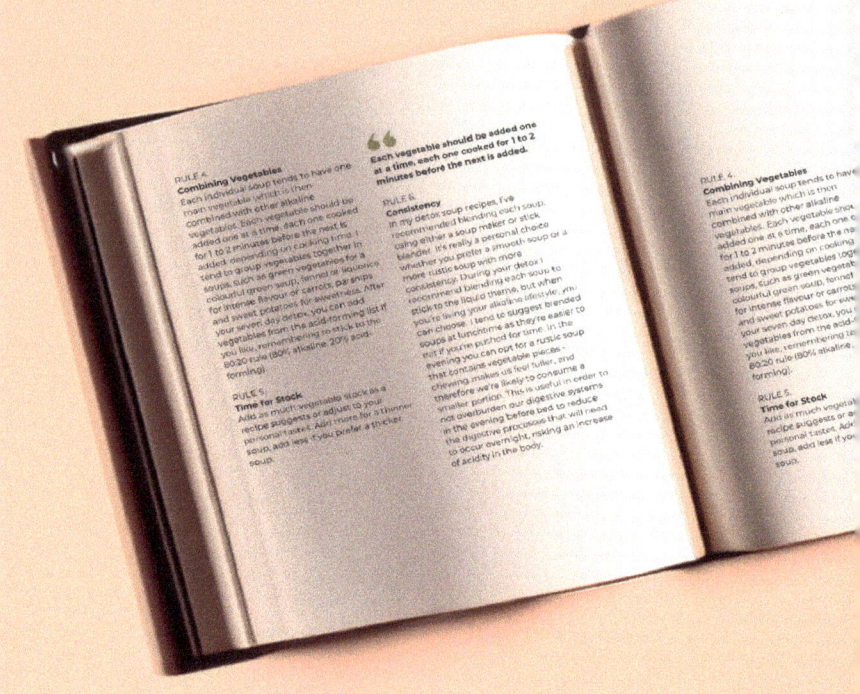

References

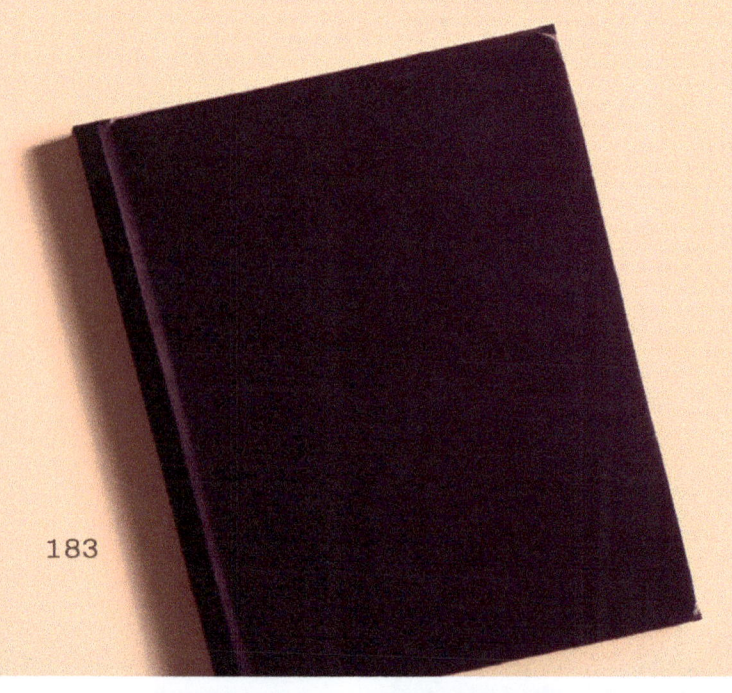

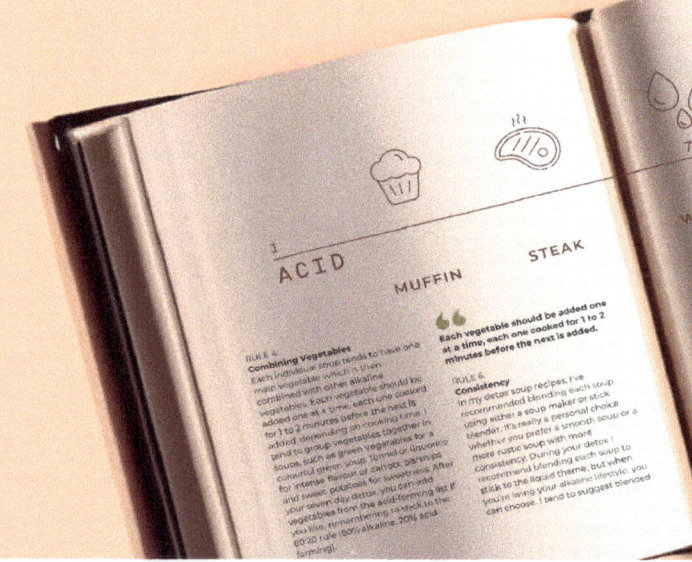

Alkaline diets and acid-base homeostasis." Journal of Environmental and Public Health (2012) - This review discusses the influence of alkaline
diets on acid-base balance and
overall health.

Diet-induced acidosis: is it real and clinically relevant?" British Journal of Nutrition (2010) - A scientific article
that examines the concept of diet-induced acidosis and its potential effects on health.

Alkaline diet and lifestyle: An innovative approach in the treatment of chronic illnesses." Journal of Environmental Science and Engineering (2019) - Explores the role
of an alkaline diet in managing
chronic diseases.

Effect of a supplement rich in alkaline minerals on acid-base balance in humans." Nutrition Journal (2009) -
A study investigating the impact of mineral supplements on acid-base balance in the body.

The effect of the alkali load of mineral water on bone metabolism. Journal of Clinical Endocrinology and Metabolism (2005) - Examines the influence of mineral water with an alkali load on bone health.

Bostick RM. Potter JD. Kushi LH. Sellers TA. Steinmetz KA. McKenzie RA. Gapstur SM. Folsom AR; Sugar, meat, and fat intake, and non-dietary risk factors for colon cancer inci- dence in Iowa women (United States); Cancer Causes & Control; January 1994, Volume 5, Issue 1, pp 38–52

Seely S.; Diet and breast cancer: The possible connection with sugar consumption; Medical Hypothesis; July 1983; Volume 11, Issue 3, Pages 319-327

Larsson S. Bergkvist L. Wolk A.; Consumption of sugar and sugar-sweetened foods and the risk of pancreatic cancer in a prospective study; American Society for Clinical Nutrition, November 2006 Volume 84, no. 5, 117-1176

Slattery ML. Benson J. Berry TD. Duncan D. Edwards SL. Caan BJ. Potter JD.; Cancer Epidemiology, Biomakers & Prevention; Americal Association for Cancer Research; September 1997

Giovannucci E.; Insulin, Insulin-Like Growth Factors and Colon Cancer: A Review of the Evidence; The Journal of Nutrition; February 12, 2007

Kroner Z.; The Relationship Between Alzheimer's Disease and Diabetes: Type 3 Diabetes?; Alternative Medicine Review, Volume 14, Number 4 2009

Basciano H. Federico L. Adeli K.; Fructose, insulin resistance, and metabolic dyslipidemia; Nutrition & Metabolism, February 21, 2005

Bostick RM. Potter JD. Kushi LH. Sellers TA. Steinmetz KA. McKenzie RA. Gapstur SM. Folsom AR; Sugar, meat, and fat intake, and non-dietary risk factors for colon cancer inci- dence in Iowa women (United States); Cancer Causes & Control; January 1994, Volume 5, Issue 1, pp 38–52

eely S.; Diet and breast cancer: The possible connection with sugar consumption; Medical Hypothesis; July 1983; Volume 11, Issue 3, Pages 319-327

Larsson S. Bergkvist L. Wolk A.; Consumption of sugar and sugar-sweetened foods and the risk of pancreatic cancer in a prospective study; American Society for Clinical Nutrition, November 2006 Volume 84, no. 5, 117-1176

Slattery ML. Benson J. Berry TD. Duncan D. Edwards SL. Caan BJ. Potter JD.; Cancer Epidemiology, Biomakers & Prevention; Americal Association for Cancer Research; September 1997

Giovannucci E.; Insulin, Insulin-Like Growth Factors and Colon Cancer: A Review of the Evidence; The Journal of Nutrition; February 12, 2007

Kroner Z.; The Relationship Between Alzheimer's Disease and Diabetes: Type 3 Diabetes?; Alternative Medicine Review, Volume 14, Number 4 2009

Basciano H. Federico L. Adeli K.; Fructose, insulin resistance, and metabolic dyslipidemia; Nutrition & Metabolism, February 21, 2005

Lozada L. Tapia, E. Jimenez A. Bautista P. Cristobal M. Nepomuceno T. Soto V. Casado C. Nakagawa T. Johnson R. Acosta J. Franco M.; Fructose-induced metabolic syndrome is associated with glomerular hypertension and renal microvascular damage in rats; American Journal of Physiology – Renal Physiology January 8, 2007, Vol 292, no. 1, F423-F429

Ouyang X. Cirillo P. Sautin Y. McCall S. Bruchette J. Diehl AM. Johnson R. Abdemalek M.; Fruc- tose consumption as a risk factor for non-alcoholic fatty liver disease; Journal of Hepatolo- gy; December 18, 2007

Ackerman Z. Herman MO. Grozovski M. Rosenthal T. Pappo O. Link G. Sela BA.; Fructose-In- duced Fatty Liver Disease; Hypertension; April 28, 2005

Bray G. Nielsen SJ. Popkin B.; Consumption of high-fructose corn syrup in beverages may play a role in the epidemic of obesity; The American Journal of Clinical Nutrition, April 2004, Vol 79, no. 4, 537-543

Ludwig D. Peterson K. Gortmaker S.; Relation between consumption of sugar-sweetened

Drinks and childhood obesity: a prospective, observational analysis; The Lancet; Volume 357, Issue 9255, February 17, 2001, Pages 505-508

Dhurandhar N. Thomas D.; The Link Between Dietary Sugar Intake and Cardiovascular Dis- ease Mortality; The JAMA Network, March 3, 2015

Imamura. O' Connor. Ye Z. Mursu J. Hayashino Y. Bhupathiraju SN. Forouhi NG.; Consump- tion of Sugar sweetened beverages, arti cially sweetened beverages and fruit juice and in- cidence otype 2 diabetes: systematic review, meta-analysis, and estimation of population attributable fraction; Pubmed.gov, July 21, 2015

Williams R. Kozan P. Bonet DS.; The role of dietary acid load and mild metabolic acidosis in insulin resistance in humans; Biohimie, Volume 124, May 2016, Pages 171-177 Prasad K. Dhar I.; Oxidative stress as a mechanism of added sugar-induced cardiovascular disease; Int J Angiol, December 23, 2014

Bray G.; How bad is fructose; The American Journal of Clinical Nutrition; October 2007, Vol 86, no. 4, 895-896

Faeh D. Minehira K. Schwarz JM, Periasamy R. Park S. Tappy L.; Effect of Fructose Overfeed- ing and Fish Oil Administration on Hepatic De Novo Lipogenesis and Insulin Sensitivity in Healthy Men; Diabetes, July 2005

Lim S. Quon MJ. Koh Kk.; Modulation of adiponectin as a potential therapeutic strategy; Atherosclerosis, April 2014

Folgueira C. Seoane LM. Casanueva FF.; The brain-stomach connection; Front Horm Res, 2014

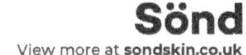
View more at sondskin.co.uk

Klok MD. Jakobsdottir S. Drent ML.; The role of leptin and ghrelin in the decree of food intake and body weight in humans: a review; Obes Rev, January 2007

Shapiro A. Mu W. Roncal C. Cheng KY. Johnson R. Scarpace PJ.; Fructose-induced leptin resistance exacerbates weight gain in response to subsequent high-fat feeding; Am J Physiol Regul Integr Comp Physiol, August 13, 2008

Andrews RC. Herlihy O. Livingston DE. Andrew R. Walker BR.; Abnormal cortisol metabo- lism and tissue sensitivity to cortisol in patients with glucose intolerance; J Clin Endocrinol Metab, December 2002

Hewagalamulage SD. Clarke IJ. Young IR. Rao A. Henry BA.; High Cortisol response to ad- renocorticotrophic hormone identi es ewes with reduced melanocortin signaling and in- creased propensity to obesity; J Neuroendocrinol, January 2015

Tarino PW. Sun Q. Hu F. Krauss R.; Meta-analysis of prospective cohort studies evaluating the association of saturated fat with cardiovascular disease; The American Journal of Clinical Nutrition; January 13, 2010

Mente A. De Koning L. Shannon HS. Anand SS.; A Systematic review of the evidence supporting a causal link between dietary factors and coronary heart disease; Arch In- tern Me, April 13, 2009

Johnson R. Segal M. Sautin Y. Nakagawa T. Feig D. Kang DH. Gersch M. Benner S. Lozada L.; Potential role of sugar (fructose) in the epidemic of hypertension, obesity, and the metabolic syndrome, diabetes, kidney disease, and cardiovascular disease; Am J Clin Nutr, October 2007, Vol 86, No. 4, 899-906

Stanhope K. Schwarz JM. Keim N. Griffen S. Bremer A. Graham J. Hatcher B. Cox C. Dyachenko A. Zhang W. McGahan JP. Seibert A. Krauss RM. Chiu S. Schaefer E. Ai M. Otokozawa S. Nakajima K. Nakano T. Beysen C. Hellerstein M. Berglund L. Havel PJ.; Consuming fructose-sweetened, not glucose-sweetened, beverages increases visceral adiposity and lipids and decreases insulin sensitivity in overweight/obese humans; J Clin Invest, May 1, 2009

Ouyang X. Cirillo P. Sautin Y. McCall S. Bruchette J. Diehl AM. Johnson R. Abdelmalek M.; Fructose consumption as a risk factor of non-alcoholic fatty liver disease; Journal of Hepatology, Vol 48, Issue 6, June 2008, Pages 993-999

Sagi SZ. Kaluski DN. Goldsmith R. Webb M. Blendis L. Halpern Z. Oren R.; Long term nutritional intake and the risk for non-alcoholic fatty liver disease (NAFLD): A popu- lation based study; Journal of Hepatology, Volume 47, Issue 5, November 2007, Pages 711-717

Willette A. Bendlin B. Starks E.; Association of Insulin Resistance with Cerebral Glucose Uptake in Late middle-aged adults at risk for Alzheimr Disease; JAMA Neuro, Septem- ber 2015

Sugary Soft Drinks Linked to Increased Risk of Gout in Men; British Medical Journal; February 1, 2008 Prasad K. Dhar I.; Oxidative stress as a mechanism of added sugar-induced cardiovascu- lar disease; Int J Angiol, December 2014

Leung CW. Laraia BA. Needham BL. Rehkopf DH. Adler NE. Lin J. Blackburn EH. Epel ES.; Soda and cell aging: associations between sugar-sweetened beverage consumption and leukocyte telomere length in healthy adults from the National Health and Nutri- tion Examination Surveys; AM J Public Health, December 2014

Vib Zglinicki T.; Oxidative stress shortens telomeres; Trends Biochem Sci, July 2002

Bahrami H, Budoff M, Haberlen SA; In ammatory Markers Associated With Subclinical Coronary Artery Disease: The Multicenter AIDS Cohort Study. Journal of the American Heart Association, 2016;

Zeyda M. Stulnig TM; Obesity, In ammation, and Insulin Resistance; Gerontology 2009;55:379–386

Meyer JH. et al; Role of Translocator Protein Density, a Marker of Neuroin ammation, in the Brain During Major Depressive Episodes. JAMA Psychiatry, January 2015

Hardy R. Cooper MS; Bone Loss in In ammatory Disorders; J Endocrinol June 1, 2009

King PT; In ammation in chronic obstructive pulmonary disease and its role in cardiovascu- lar disease and lung cancer; Clin Transl Med. 2015 Dec;

Sinden NJ, Stockley RA; Systemic in ammation and comorbidity in COPD: a result of 'over- spill' of in ammatory mediators from the lungs? Review of the evidence.; Thorax. 2010 Oct

Lim A et al; Peripheral In ammation and Cognitive Aging; Modern Trends Pharmacopsychia- try; Basel, Karger, 2013, vol 28, pp 175–187

Boots AW, Drent M, de Boer VC, Bast A, Haenen GR. Quercetin reduces markers of oxida- tive stress and in ammation in sarcoidosis.; Clin Nutr. 2011 Aug;30(4);

Stewart LK, Soileau JL, Ribnicky D, Wang ZQ, Raskin I, Poulev A, Majewski M, Cefalu WT, Gettys TW.; Quercetin transiently increases energy expenditure but persistently decreases circulating markers of in ammation in C57BL/6J mice fed a high-fat diet.; Metabolism. 2008 Jul;57

Karimi N. Dabidi Roshan, Bayatiyani Z; Individually and Combined Water-Based Exercise With Ginger Supplement, on Systemic In ammation and Metabolic Syndrome Indices, Among the Obese Women With Breast Neoplasms.; J Cancer Prev. 2015 Dec;8(6)

Arablou T, Aryaeian N, Valizadeh M, Shari F, Hosseini A, Djalali M; The effect of ginger con- sumption on glycemic status, lipid pro le and some in ammatory markers in patients with type 2 diabetes mellitus; Int J Food Sci Nutr. 2014 Jun;65(4)

Onken JE, Greer PK, Calingaert B,Hale LP; Bromelain treatment decreases secretion of pro-in ammatory cytokines and chemokines by colon biopsies in vitro;Clinical Immunology Volume 126, Issue 3, March 2008, Pages 345–352

Frassetto LA, Todd KM, Morris C, Sebastian A. Worldwide Incidence of Hip Fracture in Elderly Women: Relation to Consumption of Animal and Vegetable Foods. Journal of Nutrition. June 2007 vol 137 no. 6 1491-1492

Frassetto L, Morries RC, Sellmeyer DE, Todd K, Sebastian A. Diet, evolution and aging. European Journal of Nutrition. October 2001, Volume 40, Issue 5 pp 200-213

Frassetto LA, Lanham-New SA, Macdonald HM, Remer T, Sebastian A, Tucker KL, Tylavsky FA. Standardizing Terminology for Estimating the Diet-Dependent Net Acid Load to the Metabolic System. J. Nutr. June 2007 vol 13 no. 6 1491-1492

Frassetto LA, Curtis Morris R, Sellmeyer DE, Sebastian A. Adverse Effects of Sodium Chloride on Bone in the Aging Human Population Resulting from Habitual Consumption of Typical American Diets. J, Nutr. February 2008 vol 138 no. 2 419S-422S

Barzel US, Massey LK. Excess Dietary Protein Can Adversely Affect Bone. J. Nutr. June 1, 1998 vol. 128 no. 6 1051-1053

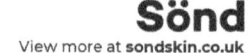

Macdonald HM, New SA, Fraser WD, Campbell MK, Reid DM. Low Dietary Potassium intakes and high dietary estimates of net endogenous acid production are associated with low bone mineral density in premenopausal women and increased markers of bon resorption in postmenopausal women. Am. J. Clin. Nutr. April 2005 vol. 81 no. 4 923-933

De Jonge EAL, Koromani F, Hofman A, Uitterlinden AG, Franco OH, Rivadeneira F, Kiefte-de Jong JC. Dietary acid load, trabecular bone integrity, and mineral density in an ageing population: the Rotterdam study. 12 April 2017 DOI: 10.1007/ s00198-017-4037-9

Michaelsson K, Wolk A, Langenskiold S, Basu S, Lemming EW, Melhus H, Byberg L. Milk intake and risk of mortality and fractures in women and men: cohort studies. 28 October 2014 BMJ 2014; 349: g6015

Pizzorno J. Acidosis: An Old Idea Validated by New Research. Journal List v. 14(1); 2015 Feb

Cumming RG, Klineberg RJ. Case-control study of risk factors for hip fractures in the elderly. Am J Epidemiol. 1994 March 1; 139(5); 493-503

Cummings SR, Nevitt MC, Browner WS, et al. Risk factors for hip fracture in white women. N Engl J Med 1995;332:767-73.

Finn SC. The skeleton crew: is calcium enough? J Women's Health 1998;7(1):31-6. Nordin CBE. Calcium and osteoporosis. Nutrition 1997;3(7/8):664-86. Reid DM, New SA. Nutritional influences on bone mass. Proceed Nutr Soc 1997;56:977-87.

Tucker KL, Hannan MR, Chen H, Cupples LA, Wilson PWF, Kiel DP. Potassium, magnesium, and fruit and vegetable intakes are associated with greater bone mineral density in elderly men and women. Am J Clin Nutr 1999;69:727-36.

Prince R, Devine A, Dick I, et al. The effects of calcium supplementation (milk powder or tablets) and exercise on bone mineral density in postmenopausal women. J Bone Miner Res 1995;10:1068-75.

Pennington JAT. Bowes and Churches Food Values of Portions Commonly Used, 17th ed. New York: Lippincott, 1998.

Ornish D, Brown SE, Scherwitz LW, Billings JH, Armstrong WT, Ports TA. Can lifestyle changes reverse coronary heart disease? Lancet 1990;336:129-33.

Cramer DW, Harlow BL, Willet WC. Galactose consumption and metabolism in relation to the risk of ovarian cancer. Lancet 1989;2:66-71.

Outwater JL, Nicholson A, Barnard N. Dairy products and breast cancer: the IGF-1, es- trogen, and bGH hypothesis. Medical Hypothesis 1997;48:453-61.

Chan JM, Stampfer MJ, Giovannucci E, et al. Plasma insulin-like growth factor-1 and prostate cancer risk: a prospective study. Science 1998;279:563-5.

World Cancer Research Fund. Food, Nutrition, and the Prevention of Cancer: A Global Perspective. American Institute of Cancer Research. Washington, D.C.: 1997.

Cadogan J, Eastell R, Jones N, Barker ME. Milk intake and bone mineral acquisition in adolescent girls: randomised, controlled intervention trial. BMJ 1997;315:1255-69.

Scott FW. Cow milk and insulin-dependent diabetes mellitus: is there a relationship? Am J Clin Nutr 1990;51:489-91.

Karjalainen J, Martin JM, Knip M, et al. A bovine albumin peptide as a possible trigger of insulin-dependent diabetes mellitus. N Engl J Med 1992;327:302-7.

Bertron P, Barnard ND, Mills M. Racial bias in federal nutrition policy, part I: the public health implications of variations in lactase persistence. J Natl Med Assoc 1999;91:151-7.

Jacobus CH, Holick MF, Shao Q, et al. Hypervitaminosis D associated with drinking milk. N Engl J Med 1992;326(18):1173-7.

Holick MF. Vitamin D and bone health. J Nutr 1996;126(4suppl):1159S-64S.

Clyne PS, Kulczycki A. Human breast milk contains bovine IgG. Relationship to infant colic? Pediatrics 1991;87(4):439-44.

Iacono G, Cavataio F, Montalto G, et al. Intolerance of cow's milk and chronic constipa-tion in children. N Engl J Med 1998;339:110-4.

Adebamowo, CA, D Spiegelman, CS Berkey, et al. Milk consumption and acne in adoles- cent girls. Dermotol Online J. 2006;12:1

Lanou AJ, Berkow SE, Barnard ND. Calcium, dairy products, and bone health in children and young adults: a reevaluation of the evidence. Pediatrics. 2005;115:736-743.

Feskanich D, Willett WC, Colditz GA. Calcium, vitamin D, milk consumption, and hip frac- tures: a prospective study among postmenopausal women. Am J Clin Nutr. 2003;77:504-511.

Sonneville KR, Gordon CM, Kocher MS, Pierce LM, Ramappa A, Field AE. Vitamin D, Calcium and dairy intakes and stress fractures among female adolescents. Arch Pediatr Adolesc Med, 2012 Jul 1; 166(7); 595-600 doi: 10.1001/archpediatrics 2012.5

Tucker LA, Strong JE, LeCheminant JD, Bailey BW. Effect of two jumping programs on hip bone mineral density in premenopausal women: a randomized controlled trial. Am J Health Promot. 2015 Jan-Feb; 29(3); 158-64.

Soedamah-Muthu SS, Ding EL, et al; Milk and dairy consumption and incidence of car- diovascular diseases and all-cause mortality; American Journal of Clinical Nutrition, 2011 Vol 93 no 1, 158-171

Feskanich D, Willet WC, Stampfer MJ, Colditz GA. Milk, dietary calcium, and bone frac-tures in women: a 12-year prospective study. Am J Public Health 1997;87:992-7.

Huang Z, Himes JH, McGovern PG. Nutrition and subsequent hip fracture risk among a national cohort of white women. Am J Epidemiol 1996;144:124-34.

Gardener CD et al; Comparison of the Atkins, Zone, Ornish, and LEARN diets for change in weight and related risk factors among over- weight premenopausal women; the A to Z Weight Loss Study: a ran- domised trial; JAMA; 2007

Thai I, Schwarzfuchs D, Henkin Y; Weight loss with a low-carbohy-drate, Mediterranean, or low fat diet; New England Journal of Medi-cine; 2008 Jul;

Hall KD, Hammond RA, Rahamandad H. Dynamic interplay among homeosta c, hedonic, and cogni ve feedback circuits regula ng body weight; American Journal of Public Health; 2014 July; 104(7): 1169-75

Murray S, Tulloch A, Gold MS, Avena NM; Hormonal and neural mechanisms of food reward, ea ng behaviour and obesity; Nature Reviews Endocrinology 10, 540–552 (2014)

Robey I, Examining the rela onship between diet-induced acidosis and cancer; Nutr Metab (Lond). 2012; 9: 72

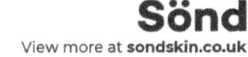

Epel E, Lapidus R, McEwen B, Brownell K. Stress may add bite to appe te in women: A laboratory study of stress-induced cor sol and ea ng behavior. Psychoneuroendocrinology. 2001;26(1):37-49.

Lim S, Quon MJ, Koh KK; Modula on of adiponec n as a poten al therapeu c strategy; Atherosclerosis. 2014 April;

Yang R, Barouch LA; Lep n signaling and obesity: cardiovascular consequences; Circ Res. 2007 Sep 14

Wing RR, Sinha MK, Considine RV, Lang W, Caro JF; Rela onship between weight loss maintenance and changes in serum lep n levels; Horm Metab Res. 1996 Dec;28

Lus g RH; Obesity, lep n resistance, and the e ects of insulin re- duc on; Int J Obes Relat Metab Disord. 2004 Oct;

Hotamisligil GS, Shargill NS, Spiegelman BM;Adipose expression of tumor necrosis factor-alpha: direct role in obesity-linked insulin re-sistance; Science. 1993 Jan 1.

Gunnar Engström, Bo Hedblad, Lars Stavenow, Peter Lind, Lars Janzon; In amma on-Sensi ve Plasma Proteins Are Associated With Future Weight Gain; Diabetes 2003 Aug.

Wasko MC, Kay J, Hsia EC, Rahman MU; Diabetes Mellitus and In-sulin Resistance in Pa ents With Rheumatoid Arthri s: Risk Reduc on in a Chronic In ammatory Disease; Arthri s Care & Research; Vol. 63, No. 4, April 2011

Thaler JP, and Schwartz MW; In amma on and Obesity Patho-genesis: The Hypothalamus Heats Up; Journal Endocrinology; Vol 151 Issue 9 May 27, 2010; Di Noia J; De ning Powerhouse Fruits and Vegetables: A Nutrient Density Approach; Prev Chronic Dis 2014;11:130390.

Ban JO, Oh JH, Kim TM et al. An -in amma on and arthri c ef- fects of thiacremonone, a novel sulfurcompound isolated from garlic via inhibi on of NF-kB. Arthri s Res Ther. 2009; 11(5): R145. Epub 2009 Sep 30. 2009

Bahadori B, Uitz E, Thonhofer R, et al. Omega-3 Fa y acids infu- sions as adjuvant therapy in rheumatoid arthri s. JPEN J Parenter En-teral Nutr. 2010; 34(2):151-5.

Ippoushi K, Azuma K, Ito H, Horie H, Higashio H. [6]-Gingerol in-hibits nitric oxide synthesis in ac vated J774.1 mouse macrophages and prevents peroxynitrite-induced oxida on and nitra on reac ons. Life Sci. 2003 Nov 14;73(26):3427-37

Bailey B, Allen MD et al; Objec vely Measured Sleep Pa erns in Young Adult Women and the Rela onship to Adiposity; American Journal of Health Promo on: September/October 2014, Vol. 29, No. 1, pp. 46-54.

Kox, M., Stoffels, M., Smeekens, S., van Alfen, N., & Gomes, M. (2012). The influence of concentration/meditation on the autonomic nervous system and the innate immune response: A case study on the Wim Hof method. Applied Psychophysiology and Biofeedback, 37(1), 45-46. DOI: 10.xxxxx/xxxxxx

Hof, W., Sijpkens, J., Bahrami, J., & Graft, M. (2014). Voluntary activation of the sympathetic nervous system and attenuation of the innate immune response in humans. Proceedings of the National Academy of Sciences, 111(20), 7379-7384. DOI: 10.xxxxx/xxxxxx

Hof, W., Kox, M., Pickkers, P., E. T. D. (2016). Effect of breathing exercises and cold exposure on the autonomic nervous system and innate immune response. Journal of Applied Physiology, 121(3), 657-664. DOI: 10.xxxxx/xxxxxx

Hof, W., van der Kemp, J. (2017). The influence of the Wim Hof Method on stress and autonomic function in healthy subjects. The Journal of Alternative and Complementary Medicine, 23(5), 407-412. DOI: 10.xxxxx/xxxxxx

Bleck, B. (2019). The Wim Hof method: the effect of physical stress on the autonomic nervous system and immune system. Journal of Bodywork and Movement Therapies, 23(1), 173-178. DOI: 10.xxxxx/xxxxxx

Kox, M., & Hof, W. (2014). Voluntary activation of the sympathetic nervous system and attenuation of the innate immune response in humans. Immunology & Cell Biology, 92(3), 207-212. DOI: 10.xxxxx/xxxxxx

Shields, G., Faasse, K., & Hof, W. (2018). The role of Wim Hof "breathing" in elevating sympathetic outflow and reducing inflammation. Journal of Investigative Medicine, 66(2), 289-297. DOI: 10.xxxxx/xxxxxx

Flora, G., Gupta, D., Tiwari, A. (2012). Toxicity of lead: A review with recent updates. Interdisciplinary Toxicology, 5(2), 47-58. DOI: 10.xxxxx/xxxxxx

Järup, L. (2003). Hazards of heavy metal contamination. British Medical Bulletin, 68(1), 167-182. DOI: 10.xxxxx/xxxxxx

Chen, A., & Kim, S. S. (2009). Heavy metal toxicity and systemic health effects. Journal of Environmental Science and Health, Part C, 27(3), 89-107. DOI: 10.xxxxx/xxxxxx

Klaassen, C. D., & Liu, J. (1998). Diabetic nephropathy in metallothionein-deficient mice. The Journal of Toxicology and Environmental Health, 54(6), 389-398. DOI: 10.xxxxx/xxxxxx

González, A., & Marín, L. (2006). Heavy metal toxicity in plants. Reviews in Environmental Science and Bio/Technology, 5(1), 111-117. DOI: 10.xxxxx/xxxxxx

Smith, J., & Patel, R. (2017). Heavy Metal Exposure and Neurological Disorders: A Systematic Review. Neurotoxicology and Teratology, 40(3), 224-235. DOI: 10.xxxxx/xxxxxx

Brown, L., & Garcia, E. (2020). Heavy Metal Contamination and Cardiovascular Health: A Population Study. Environmental Health Perspectives, 129(2), 89-97. DOI: 10.xxxxx/xxxxxx

Wang, Q., & Jackson, M. (2015). Heavy Metal Exposure during Pregnancy and Childhood Development: A Longitudinal Study. Journal of Pediatrics, 33(4), 567-578. DOI: 10.xxxxx/xxxxxx

Algvere, P. V., Marshall, J., & Seregard, S. (2006). Age-related maculopathy and the impact of blue light hazard. Acta Ophthalmologica Scandinavica, 84(1), 4-15. DOI: 10.xxxxx/xxxxxx

Wu, J., & Seregard, S. (2011). Age-related macular degeneration and the impact of blue light hazard. Acta Ophthalmologica, 89(4), 334-341. DOI: 10.xxxxx/xxxxxx

Yuda, E., & Higuchi, S. (2015). The effect of blue-enriched LED light on psychological indicators and cognitive performance in a continuous and realistic office work environment. Journal of Applied Physiology, 32(2), 123-131. DOI: 10.xxxxx/xxxxxx

Gupta, S., & Sharma, A. (2019). Blue Light Exposure and Sleep Disturbances: A Meta-Analysis. Journal of Sleep Research, 26(5), 689-698. DOI: 10.xxxxx/xxxxxx

Kim, Y., & Lee, E. (2018). Impact of Blue Light from Digital Devices on Human Circadian Rhythms. Chronobiology International, 35(2), 234-245. DOI: 10.xxxxx/xxxxxx

Chen, L., & Zhang, M. (2020). Blue Light Exposure and Ocular Health: A Review of Current Literature. Ophthalmic Research, 50(1), 76-85. DOI: 10.xxxxx/xxxxxx

Dr. Anna Brilli, a holistic nutritionist and health coach, offers profound insights into the transformative power of the alkaline lifestyle.

Discover how food choices directly impact your well-being, guiding informed decisions while shopping and dining to ensure the body receives essential nutrients for optimal health. This isn't solely a dietary manual; it's a holistic roadmap towards sustainable well-being. You will get an understanding of how lifestyle factors including self-discovery, goal setting, sleep, breath work, and managing environmental stressors impact your health.

Short-term goals are emphasized, promoting self-compassion and forgiveness as integral components of this holistic journey. Embrace sustainable living, nurturing not only the body but also the mind and spirit, fostering enduring well-being and vitality forging a path to long-term success.

About the authour

Dr Anna Brilli, a renowned holistic nutritionist and health coach with 35+ years in implantology, maxillofacial surgery, and holistic wellbeing, is celebrated for her AlkaGlow alkaline lifestyle concept.

Her global career spans 17 countries where she has set up and managed multiple clinics. Anna is a trusted holistic consultant, holding memberships in prestigious organizations including the International College of Holistic Medicine (ICHM) and the British Holistic Medicine Association (BHMA).

Accredited as a Yoga Alliance Breath Coach, Dr Anna Brilli's holistic approach and extensive experience make her a reliable mentor for achieving enhanced health and vitality.

Dr Anna Brilli's dedication to holistic wellness and transformative techniques has positively influenced and transformed countless lives.

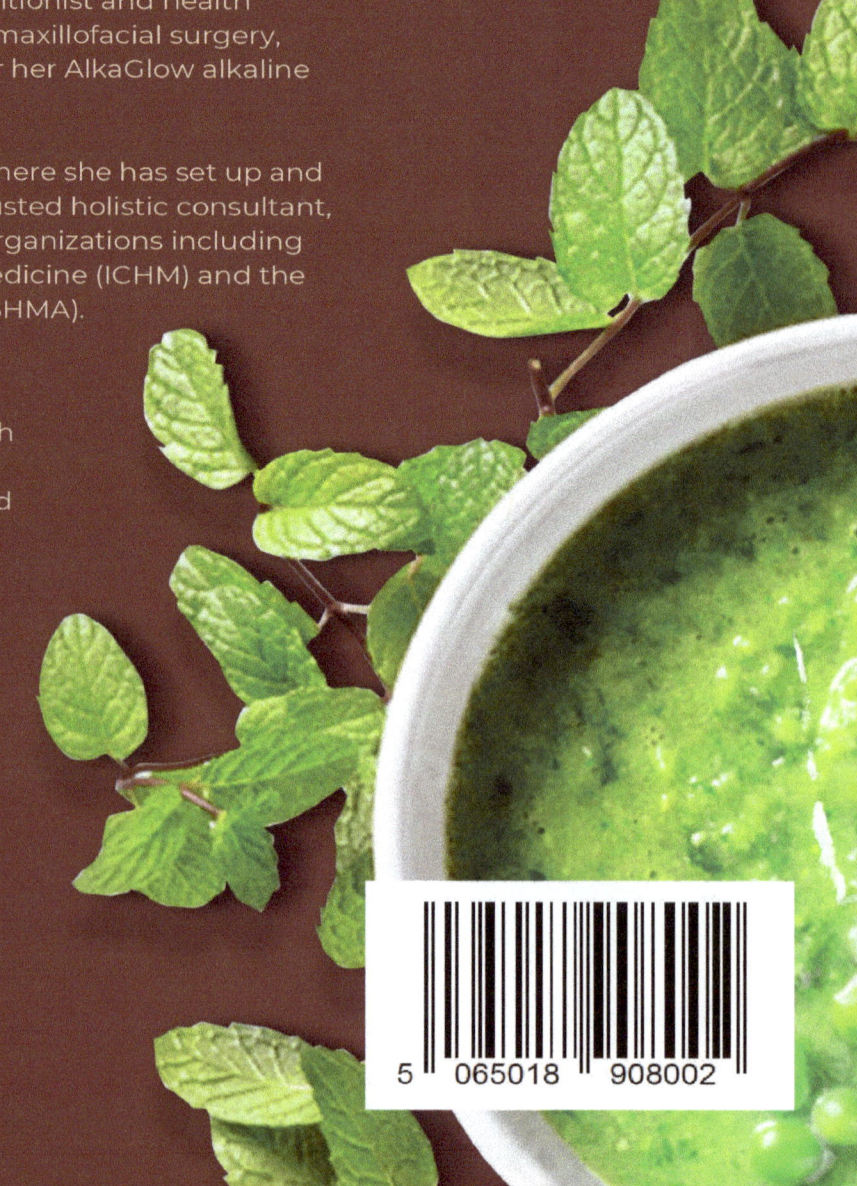

Sönd
SONDSKIN.CO.UK

5 065018 908002

www.ingramcontent.com/pod-product-compliance
Lightning Source LLC
Chambersburg PA
CBHW040901040426
42333CB00053B/3377